DR. BARBARA O'NEILL'S COOKBOOK

Easy Recipes, Nutritional Guidance, Healthy Eating, Plant-Based Meals, Simple Cooking Tips, and Wellness for a Vibrant Life

Dr. Chris G. Jayden

COPYRIGHT © 2024 BY DR. CHRIS G. JAYDEN

CHAPTER ONE
INTRODUCTION TO HOLISTIC NUTRITION

The holistic perspective on nutrition is a comprehensive method of feeding that emphasizes the relationship between the body, mind, and spirit. It highlights how crucial it is to eat complete, unprocessed foods in order to support general health and wellbeing. Holistic nutrition considers a variety of aspects, including lifestyle, emotional well-being, and environmental impacts, in contrast to traditional nutrition, which frequently concentrates only on the nutritional value of food.

Comprehending Holistic Nutrition

Fundamentally, holistic nutrition acknowledges that each person is distinct and, as such, has distinctive dietary needs. It considers the foods consumed as well as their cultivation, preparation, and consumption methods. In addition to recommending a diet low in processed foods, artificial additives, and toxins, holistic dietitians frequently support a diet high in organic fruits and vegetables, whole grains, lean meats, and healthy fats.

The Advantages of a Holistic Diet

The emphasis on preventative health measures that comes with using a holistic eating approach is one of its main advantages. Through the consumption of nutrient-dense foods and abstaining from dangerous substances, people can lessen their chance of developing chronic illnesses including diabetes, heart disease, and obesity. Holistic nutrition can also support stronger immune system performance, higher mental clarity, increased energy, and better digestion.

The Health and Wellness Philosophy of Barbara O'Neill

Well-known for her comprehensive approach to health and wellness, Barbara O'Neill is a holistic health practitioner and educator. Her guiding principle is that harmony and balance in all spheres of life—physical, mental, emotional, and spiritual—are the keys to achieving true health. O'Neill highlights the significance of paying attention to the body's inherent wisdom and showing it kindness and respect. She promotes a healthy diet, frequent exercise, stress reduction methods, and spiritual activities as part of an all-encompassing lifestyle.

The Effects of Nutrition on General Well-Being

One of the most important factors affecting general well-being is nutrition. Our bodies require certain critical elements from the food we eat in order to function correctly and sustain optimal health. A diet deficient in vital nutrients can result in inadequacies, compromised immunity, and heightened vulnerability to disease. Conversely, a well-balanced diet high in antioxidants, phytonutrients, vitamins, and minerals can promote mental clarity, emotional stability, physical vigor, and spiritual development.

Including the Mind-Body Link in Eating Behavior

Being aware of what, when, and how we eat is essential to incorporating the mind-body link into eating patterns. It involves paying attention to our bodies' signals of hunger and fullness as well as our emotional and psychological cues in order to make nourishing decisions that promote general wellbeing. This could entail using mindful eating strategies like slowing down, enjoying every bite, and observing the physical, mental, and emotional effects of various foods.

We can develop a stronger sense of awareness, connection, and harmony within ourselves and with the environment around us by adopting a holistic approach to diet. In the end, holistic nutrition is about how we fuel our body, mind, and spirit to grow and prosper in all facets of life, not simply about what we eat.

The Basics of a Well-Diet

The foundation of total wellbeing is a good diet, which supplies the vital nutrients needed to sustain physical processes, sustain energy levels, and fend off illness. The cornerstones of a nutritious diet consist of complete, nutrient-dense foods that are prioritized together with moderation and balance. People can develop eating habits that support optimum health and vitality by realizing the significance of whole foods, nutrient-dense ingredients, macronutrient balance, micronutrients, and water.

The Value of Complete Foods

Whole foods are as near to their natural state as possible, with very little processing or refining. They consist of lean proteins, healthy fats, fruits, vegetables, whole grains, legumes, nuts, and seeds. Whole foods are abundant in vital elements including vitamins, minerals, fiber, and antioxidants, in contrast to processed foods, which can have extra sugars, harmful fats, and artificial additives. Eating a diet rich in whole foods gives the body the components it needs to function at its best and promotes many internal processes, such as metabolism, digestion, immunological response, and cellular repair.

Ingredients Packed with Nutrients for Optimal Health

The concentration of nutrients in a food in relation to its calorie amount is referred to as its nutritional density. Foods high in vitamins, minerals, antioxidants, and phytonutrients per serving are referred to as nutrient-dense foods; they also lack added calories, sweets, or bad fats. Leafy greens, vibrant veggies, berries, whole grains, lean proteins, nuts, seeds, and fatty fish are a few examples of foods high in nutrients. Nutrient-dense foods should be prioritized in the diet in order to guarantee that people are getting the nutrients they need while also promoting general health and wellbeing.

Maintaining Equilibrium Macronutrients: Glucose, Proteins, and Fats

Carbohydrates, proteins, and fats are the three primary food components known as macronutrients. They are necessary for healthy physical function and generate energy. Consuming the proper amounts of each macronutrient is necessary to sustain energy levels, preserve muscle mass, control metabolism, and encourage fullness. The body uses carbohydrates, which are present in meals like fruits, vegetables, whole grains, and legumes, as its main energy source. Proteins are found in foods including meat, chicken, fish, eggs, dairy, legumes, and tofu and are essential for immunological response, tissue repair, and hormone synthesis. Fats are present in foods like avocados, nuts, seeds, olive oil, and fatty seafood and are crucial for hormone production, brain function, and nutrient absorption. To guarantee that the body gets the nutrients it needs to function at its best, a balanced diet consists of a range of foods high in macronutrients.

Micronutrients: Vital Minerals and Vitamins for Good Health

Micronutrients are vitamins and minerals that the body needs for a number of physiological functions, such as immune system response, metabolism, bone health, and antioxidant defense. Micronutrients are essential for maintaining general health and wellbeing, even though they are needed in smaller quantities than macronutrients. Vitamins A, C, D, E, K, B vitamins, calcium, magnesium, iron, zinc, selenium, and potassium are a few examples of micronutrients. Numerous foods, such as fruits, vegetables, whole grains, dairy products, meat, poultry, fish, nuts, and seeds, are rich sources of these nutrients. A diverse and balanced diet that includes a wide variety of vibrant fruits and vegetables will guarantee that you are getting enough of the vital micronutrients your body needs to function at its best.

Hydration: The Benefits of Water for Health

Water is necessary for life and is involved in many body processes, such as regulating body temperature, transporting nutrients, eliminating waste, lubricating joints, and supplying water to cells. Drinking enough water throughout the day is something that many people forget to do, despite the fact that staying well hydrated is essential for general health and wellbeing. The amount of water that should be consumed each day varies based on age, gender, activity level, and climate, but as a general rule of thumb, you should aim to drink at least eight 8-ounce glasses. Apart from drinking plain water, there are additional options to stay hydrated, like herbal teas, infused water, fruits, and vegetables. Maintaining proper hydration is crucial for boosting digestive health, improving skin tone, and advancing general wellness in addition to maximizing physical and mental performance.

In summary, the cornerstones of a healthy diet are based on the ideas that complete, nutrient-dense foods are important and that moderation and balance are important. People can develop eating habits that support optimum health, vitality, and longevity by include whole foods, nutrient-dense items, balanced macronutrients, critical micronutrients, and adequate hydration in their diet.

CHAPTER TWO

PLANT-BASED DIET FOR HEALTHFUL VIBRANT LIVING

A diet high in fruits, vegetables, whole grains, legumes, nuts, and seeds has been linked to several health benefits, which has led to a rise in the popularity of plant-based eating in recent years. Adopting a plant-based diet entails giving plant-based foods first priority while reducing or giving up animal items. People can get vital nutrients, such as protein, fiber, vitamins, minerals, and antioxidants, to support vibrant health and general well-being by constructing balanced meals with a range of plant-based components. Making the switch to a plant-based diet may seem overwhelming at first, but with the right preparation and knowledge, it can be a fulfilling and long-term approach to nourish the body and safeguard the environment.

Adopting a Plant-Based Diet

Adopting a plant-based diet entails changing the emphasis of meals from animal products to plant-based foods. Fruits, vegetables, whole grains, legumes, nuts, seeds, and plant-based substitutes for dairy, meat, and eggs can all fall under this category. Plant-based eating is more about including more plant-based foods in one's meals and snacks than it is about strictly adhering to a particular diet. A plant-based diet is popular among people for a variety of reasons, such as health, animal welfare, environmental sustainability, and cultural or religious convictions. Plant-based diet is a healthful and sustainable method to fuel the body because it places an emphasis on whole, unprocessed foods that are high in nutrients and devoid of artificial additives, preservatives, and trans fats.

Creating Balanced Meals Devoid of Animal Ingredients

To ensure optimal intake of key nutrients, a range of plant-based components must be used when building balanced meals devoid of animal products. To maintain optimum health and energy levels, each meal should include a combination of carbohydrates, proteins, healthy fats, vitamins, minerals, and fiber. Foods high in carbohydrates, such as whole grains, legumes, fruits, and vegetables, give the body energy and fiber to aid in digestion and satiety. Nuts, seeds, quinoa, beans, lentils, tofu, tempeh, seitan, edamame, and other plant foods high in protein supply the essential amino acids required for hormone production, immunological response, and muscle repair. Essential fatty acids are found in healthy fats from foods like avocados, nuts, seeds, olive oil, and coconut oil. These fats assist hormone balance, nutrition absorption, and brain health. People can make satisfying, well-balanced plant-based meals that support general health by including a range of plant foods into their meals and snacks.

Plant Foods High in Protein for Long-Term Energy

Protein is a vital ingredient that the body needs for many physiological processes, such as immune system function, muscle repair, hormone generation, and enzyme functioning. Although many people think of animal products as the main source of protein, there are many of plant meals that are high in protein and can provide sufficient amounts to promote vigor and health. Plant foods high in protein include quinoa, almonds, seeds, nut butters, legumes, chickpeas, tofu, tempeh, seitan, edamame, and plant-based protein powders. These foods are easy to include in meals and snacks to maintain sustained energy levels and muscle recovery since they include critical amino acids required for protein synthesis. To support general health and well-being, people can meet their protein demands and ensure they get all the essential amino acids by including a range of plant foods high in protein in their diet.

Fiber's Advantages for Plant-Based Diets

Plant-based meals contain fiber, a type of carbohydrate that is vital for heart health, blood sugar regulation, weight control, and digestive health. Because plant-based diets are rich in fruits, vegetables, whole grains, legumes, nuts, and seeds, they are inherently high in fiber. Dietary fiber helps maintain a healthy gut microbiota, encourages regularity, reduces constipation, and gives the stool more volume. In addition to stabilizing blood sugar and lowering cholesterol, soluble fiber also increases sensations of fullness and satisfaction. Insoluble fiber encourages bowel regularity, prevents constipation, and gives the stool more volume. People can support digestive health, maintain a healthy weight, lower their chance of developing chronic diseases, and enhance their general well-being by eating a plant-based diet high in fiber.

Advice for Making the Switch to a Plant-Based Diet

Making the switch to a plant-based diet can be an exciting and fulfilling experience, but for some people, there may be obstacles to overcome. The following advice will help to ensure a more seamless and sustainable transition:

1.Start slowly: Increase the amount of plant-based meals and snacks in your diet at first, then progressively cut back on the amount of animal products you eat. To find tasty and fulfilling plant-based meals, try out different recipes, ingredients, and cooking techniques.

2.Give whole, unprocessed plant foods like fruits, vegetables, whole grains, legumes, nuts, and seeds priority. These nutrient-dense, fiber- and antioxidant-rich foods can serve as the cornerstone of a plant-based diet.

3.Explore a range of plant-based protein sources, including quinoa, almonds, seeds, seitan, edamame, beans, lentils, and chickpeas. You can also experiment with plant-based protein powders. These items are plenty of protein and can be incorporated into a lot of different recipes to make tasty and filling meals.

4.Be aware of your nutrient needs: Monitor the amount of nutrients you eat to make sure you are getting enough protein, iron, calcium, vitamin B12, omega-3 fatty acids, and other vital nutrients for your body. To support optimal health, think about include fortified meals or supplements as needed.

5.Make a plan: Give your meals and snacks some thought to make sure you have a range of plant-based options available all week. Keep a supply of basic items in your pantry, such as grains, beans, nuts, seeds, and spices. You may also make meals and snacks in bulk for quick grab-and-go options.

6.In the kitchen, use your imagination to create new and interesting plant-based meals by experimenting with flavors, textures, and cuisines. Explore new plant-based recipes, ingredients, and cooking methods to find nourishing and tasty meals that you enjoy.

7.Pay attention to how different foods make you feel on a physical, mental, and emotional level. Listen to your body. Take note of how your food affects your mood, digestion, energy levels, and general well-being, and adapt as necessary to maintain your health and vitality.

To sum up, eating a plant-based diet has many health advantages and can be a tasty, fulfilling, and environmentally friendly method to fuel the body and save the environment. People can support vibrant health and overall well-being for themselves and future generations by adopting a plant-based lifestyle, creating balanced meals with a variety of plant-based ingredients, adding plant foods high in protein for sustained energy, enjoying the benefits of fiber in plant-based diets, and following advice for making the switch to a plant-based diet.

Creating Healthful Dinners using Whole Foods

Creating wholesome meals from whole foods is a fundamental part of using diet to support health and vitality. Whole foods serve as the foundation for healthful and filling meals since they are little processed or refined while maintaining their original flavors and nutrients. People can make sure they get a wide range of nutrients, such as vitamins, minerals, antioxidants, fiber, and phytonutrients, to support general well-being by including a variety of whole foods into their meals. The options for preparing tasty and nourishing meals that satisfy the body and please the senses are numerous, ranging from whole grains and colorful vegetables to plant-powered proteins, nuts, seeds, herbs, and spices.

Whole Grain Delight: Preparing Quinoa, Brown Rice, and Other Whole Grains

A balanced diet must include whole grains because they are a great source of complex carbohydrates, fiber, protein, vitamins, and minerals. Adding a range of whole grains to meals enhances their flavor, texture, and nutritional content while encouraging fullness and steady energy levels. Nutritious whole grains such as quinoa, brown rice, barley, oats, millet, farro, bulgur, and wheat berries can be included into a variety of dishes, such as pilafs, stir-fries, soups, and morning porridges. Whole grains are easy to cook; you can cook them until they're mushy and fluffy on the stovetop, in a rice cooker, or in an Instant Pot with water or broth. Whole grain deliciousness enhances general health and well-being by giving meals more richness and nutrition.

Bright Vegetables: Adding a Trio of Colors to Your Plate

With an abundance of vitamins, minerals, antioxidants, fiber, and other nutrients to promote optimum health and vigor, vegetables are nature's nutritional powerhouses. A rainbow of vibrant vegetables can be added to meals to enhance flavor, visual appeal, and nutritional diversity. It also encourages a diet that is well-balanced and nutrient-rich. There are a gazillion ways to creatively and delectably include vegetables into meals, ranging from leafy greens and cruciferous vegetables to root vegetables, peppers, tomatoes, mushrooms, and more. Veggies improve the flavor and nutritional value of food by adding freshness, crunch, and brightness whether they are cooked in a stir-fry, sautéed, roasted, or steamed state. Accepting the bounty of colorful vegetables guarantees a diet high in nutrients that satisfies the body and promotes general health.

Plant-Powered Proteins: Tofu, Tempeh, and Legumes in Recipes

A plant-based diet must include plant-powered proteins because they offer vital amino acids, vitamins, minerals, and fiber to support immune system function, hormone production, muscle repair, and general health. Legumes are a great source of plant-based protein and may be used in a wide range of meals, including salads, burgers, dips, and soups. Examples of legumes include beans, lentils, chickpeas, and peas. Additionally high in protein, tofu, tempeh, edamame, and seitan can be utilized in a variety of recipes, such as bowls, stir-fries, curries, and sandwiches. For those looking to increase the amount of plant-based foods in their diet, plant-powered proteins are a tasty and fulfilling addition to meals because of their adaptability, flavor, and nutritional value.

Nuts and Seeds: Including Protein and Vitamins in Your Food

Nuts and seeds are a great complement to a balanced diet since they are nutrient-dense foods full of protein, healthy fats, vitamins, minerals, and antioxidants. Nuts and seeds enhance meals with texture, flavor, and nutritional content. They also help with heart health and satiety. Some of the nuts that can be eaten raw, roasted, or in nut butter form as snacks or as toppings for salads, oats, yogurt, and desserts are almonds, walnuts, pecans, cashews, pistachios, and peanuts. Similar to this, you may add seeds to salads, smoothies, yogurt bowls, baking, cooking, and raw snacks. Some examples of seeds are chia seeds, flaxseeds, hemp seeds, pumpkin seeds, and sunflower seeds. Nuts and seeds improve the flavor and nutritional value of food by adding crunch, richness, and nutrients.

Using Herbs, Spices, and Natural Sweeteners to Create Savory and Sweet Flavors

Herbs, spices, and natural sweeteners are staples in creating savory, filling dishes that satiate the palate and uplift the spirits. Spices like cinnamon, cumin, turmeric, paprika, and ginger lend depth, warmth, and complexity to food, while herbs like basil, cilantro, parsley, mint, and dill give it a fresh, fragrant touch. By experimenting with different herb and spice combinations, people may develop flavor profiles that are both distinctive and tasty, elevating their meals to new levels. Furthermore, you can sweeten food without using refined sugar or artificial sweeteners by using natural sweeteners like dates, honey, coconut sugar, and maple syrup. People can improve general health and well-being while also improving the taste and nutritional content of their meals by embracing savory and sweet flavors with herbs, spices, and natural sweeteners.

To sum up, preparing wholesome meals using whole foods is essential to boosting vitality and health through nutrition. There are countless options for preparing tasty and nutritious meals that satisfy the senses and nourish the body, from colorful vegetables and entire grains to plant-powered proteins, nuts, seeds, herbs, and spices. People may make sure they get a wide range of nutrients to support general well-being and reap the many advantages of a balanced and nutrient-dense diet by include a variety of whole foods into their meals.

CHAPTER THREE
EATING TO STAY VITAL: RECIPES AND MEAL PLANS

Consuming nutrient-dense meals that promote energy, vitality, and general well-being is the goal of eating for vitality. People can provide their bodies with the nourishment they require to flourish by organizing meals that are balanced and include a range of healthful foods. There are countless possibilities to prepare tasty and healthy meals that support vitality and health, from weekday meal plans and weekend wellness indulgences to on-the-go snacks, family-friendly faves, and special occasion feasts.

Weekly Meal Plan: Well-Proportioned Lunches, Dinners, and Breakfasts

A weekday meal plan guarantees that people get a range of nutrients to maintain energy levels, mental clarity, and general health. It also offers structure and direction for fueling the body throughout the week. Wholesome breakfasts, filling lunches, and hearty dinners that feature an assortment of whole grains, lean proteins, healthy fats, and vibrant fruits and vegetables are all part of a well-rounded weekday meal plan. An example of a weekday menu:

• For breakfast, try overnight oats with sliced almonds, mixed berries, and honey drizzled on top.

• Quinoa salad with avocado, cucumber, cherry tomatoes, chickpeas, and lemon-tahini dressing for lunch

• Supper is baked salmon served with quinoa pilaf, steamed broccoli, and roasted sweet potatoes.

People may make weekday meals easier and guarantee they have nourishing options available all week long by planning balanced meals in advance and prepping items.

Weekend Well-Being: Snacky But Satisfying Dinners and Brunches

Weekends are meant to be spent lounging and indulging, but they can also be used to fuel the body with healthful, filling meals that promote general wellbeing. Weekend wellness meals combine healthy foods that nurture the body and the soul, striking a balance between enjoyment and nutrition. An example of a wellness menu for the weekend:

• For brunch, try whole grain pancakes with mixed berries, Greek yogurt, and maple syrup drizzled on top.

• Dinner consists of quinoa pilaf, mixed green salad, and balsamic vinaigrette paired with grilled veggie and tofu skewers.

Weekend wellbeing dinners may be decadent and filling, promoting health and vitality by combining nutrient-dense foods with aromatic herbs and spices.

Portable & Packed with Nutrients Snacks for on-the-Go

For people who lead busy lives and require quick and portable snacks to keep their bodies fueled throughout the day, on-the-go snacks are a useful option. Snacks high in nutrients offer long-lasting energy and boost concentration and productivity. Examples of quick snack ideas:

• Almond butter paired with apple slices

• Trail mix with dried fruit, nuts, and seeds

• Fresh berries and oats paired with Greek yogurt

• Sticks of veggies and hummus

• Energy balls consisting of cocoa powder, almonds, and dates

People can prevent themselves from reaching for harmful options and instead fuel their bodies with nutrient-dense foods that support vitality and well-being by planning ahead of time and keeping nutritious snacks on hand.

Family-Friendly Favorites: Kid-Approved Meals for Healthier Eating

Healthy selections that appeal to adults and kids alike make mealtimes fun and stress-free for the entire family. These are known as family-friendly meals. Meals that are appropriate for children include well-known tastes and components that appeal to young palates while still offering vital nutrients for development and growth. Family-friendly favorites include:

• Veggie-packed quesadillas with black beans, bell peppers, onions, and cheese;

• Whole wheat pasta with marinara sauce, lean mince turkey, and steamed broccoli.

• Mixed green salad and baked chicken tenders served with sweet potato fries

Parental involvement in meal planning and preparation, together with providing a range of nutrient-dense options, can help promote healthy eating habits and enhance the general health and wellbeing of the family.

Special Occasion Feasts: Festive Recipes for Joyful Get-Togethers

Festive gatherings are made more joyful and connected when delectable and sumptuous dishes are served at special occasion feasts. Even though meals for special occasions could be more decadent than meals for regular consumption, they can nevertheless contain healthy elements that promote vitality and wellbeing. An example menu for a feast fit for a memorable occasion:

• Starter: Caprese skewers topped with cherry tomatoes, fresh mozzarella, basil leaves, and balsamic glaze

• Main Course: Whole wheat dinner rolls, mashed sweet potatoes, green bean almondine, and herb-roasted turkey with cranberry sauce

• Dark chocolate avocado mousse topped with whipped cream and delicious berries for dessert

Special occasion feasts may be both joyous and health-promoting, encouraging vitality and well-being during festive gatherings by adding nutrient-dense ingredients and fragrant herbs and spices.

In summary, creating well-balanced meals and incorporating a range of complete foods into regular eating routines are essential components of eating for vitality. There are countless ways to fuel the body with nutrient-dense foods that support energy, vitality, and general well-being, from weekday meal plans and weekend wellness indulgences to on-the-go snacks, family-friendly faves, and special occasion feasts. People may provide their bodies with the nutrition they require to flourish and lead vibrant, healthy lives by emphasizing nutritious foods and tasty dishes.

Cooking Methods for Taste and Health

Cooking methods are essential for turning uncooked ingredients into tasty, nutrient-dense meals. People can promote health and well-being while improving the taste, texture, and nutritional value of their food by learning different cooking techniques. Every cooking method, including baking, grilling, and sautéing, has special advantages for producing mouthwatering, wholesome meals that please the palate and the body.

Sauteing and Steaming: Boosting Flavors and Preserving Nutrients

The delicate cooking methods of steaming and sautéing improve the flavor and texture of food while retaining its natural nutrients and flavors. Food is cooked by subjecting it to steam, either in a covered pot with a little amount of water or in a steamer basket. This technique preserves the original colors and flavors of vegetables, seafood, and poultry while aiding in the retention of water-soluble vitamins and minerals. On the other hand, sautéing is rapidly frying food over high heat in a tiny amount of oil or fat so that taste can emerge through caramelization and browning. Sautéing adds depth and richness to food while preserving the texture and nutrition of foods by using little additional fat and cooking it fast.

Baking and Roasting: Nutritious Techniques for Tasty Outcomes

Dry-heat cooking methods like roasting and baking maintain the nutritional value of ingredients while yielding mouthwatering, aromatic outcomes. Baking is the process of cooking food in an oven at a moderate temperature utilizing dry heat, which permits uniform cooking and browning without overcharring or burning. This technique is frequently used to bake cakes, bread, pastries, and casseroles. In contrast, roasting is cooking food at a higher temperature in the oven, which encourages browning and caramelization to provide rich, nuanced flavors. Vegetables, meats, birds, and fish may all be roasted to create delicate, tasty dinners that are ideal for entertaining and family get-togethers.

Adding Char and Complexity to Your Dishes with Grilling and Broiling

High-heat cooking methods like grilling and broiling give food a smokey, charred flavor while also encouraging caramelization and browning. Grilling gives foods including meats, poultry, seafood, and vegetables a unique smoky flavor and charred surface by cooking them over an open flame or hot coals. Contrarily, broiling entails cooking food in an oven at direct heat, yielding results comparable to grilling but with less exposure to smoke and flames. Both grilling and broiling are quick and easy cooking techniques that yield tasty and fulfilling meals that are guaranteed to impress. They're ideal for weeknight dinners, outdoor get-togethers, and special events.

Using Fermented and Raw Foods to Unleash the Power of Living Nutrient

Fermented and raw foods are uncooked or barely processed foods high in beneficial bacteria, live enzymes, and other bioactive substances that support vigor and health. Vitamins, minerals, antioxidants, and phytonutrients found in raw foods like fruits, vegetables, nuts, seeds, and sprouts assist healthy digestion, immunity, and general wellbeing. Fermentation is the process by which beneficial bacteria and yeast break down carbohydrates to produce fermented foods like yogurt, kefir, sauerkraut, kimchi, tempeh, and miso. Probiotics, which aid in digestion, immune system support, and gut health, are abundant in fermented foods, as are other nutrients including vitamins, minerals, and amino acids. People can use living nutrition to support their health and vitality by including raw and fermented foods in their meals and snacks.

Selecting and Using Nutritious Fats and Oils in Your Cooking

A balanced diet must include healthy fats and oils because they include vital fatty acids, fat-soluble vitamins, and other elements that are critical for optimum health and wellbeing. To enhance general wellbeing, lower inflammation, and strengthen heart health, it's critical to select and use healthy fats and oils in cooking. Nuts, seeds, avocado, coconut, olive, and fatty fish like mackerel and salmon are a few examples of healthful fats and oils. Monounsaturated and polyunsaturated fats, which are abundant in these fats and oils, have been demonstrated to lower cholesterol, lower the risk of heart disease, and promote brain function. It's crucial to use high-quality fats and oils sparingly when cooking in order to prevent consuming too many calories. In addition, cooking techniques like roasting, baking, sautéing, and steaming can reduce the need for additional fats and oils while still yielding tasty and nourishing food.

To sum up, cooking methods are essential in converting uncooked materials into scrumptious and nourishing meals that enhance health and wellbeing. Every cooking technique, such as baking, grilling, and sautéing, has special advantages for boosting the flavor, texture, and nutritional content of food. Through the acquisition of culinary skills and the selection of premium ingredients, people can prepare savory and filling meals that satiate the palate and body while promoting energy and general well-being.

FAQs and Responses

A healthy lifestyle may raise a number of concerns about nutrition, food, and general wellbeing. By answering these commonly asked questions (FAQs), people who want to make educated decisions about their health can receive helpful advice and assistance. Each topic provides insight into common concerns and problems faced on the path to better health, ranging from indulging in desserts to managing food allergies, meal prep tactics, budget-friendly eating, dining out, and the influence of stress on digestion and health.

I'm on a healthy diet; may I still have dessert?

Desserts are fine to have as part of a balanced diet, but moderation and thoughtful eating are key. Rather than regularly consuming sugary, high-calorie snacks, choose healthier substitutes that both satiate your sweet taste and offer nutritional advantages. Some instances are fruit-based sweets like fruit salad, baked apples, or "nice cream" prepared from frozen bananas combined with a small amount of milk or plant-based milk. Additionally, you can experiment with better baking substitutes like whole grain flours, honey or maple syrup, and dark chocolate, along with other wholesome components like nuts and seeds. As part of a healthy and balanced diet, you can eat dessert guilt-free by substituting wisely and paying attention to portion proportions.

How Do I Handle Sensitivities or Allergies to Food?

It's important to pay close attention to ingredient labels, meal preparation techniques, and any cross-contamination hazards when managing food allergies or sensitivities. It's crucial to speak with a healthcare provider if you think you may have a food sensitivity or allergy so they can properly diagnose and treat you. Once you are aware of the foods to stay away from, you can take precautions to reduce exposure and avoid negative reactions. When dining out, this may entail asking questions about ingredients and preparation techniques, closely reading ingredient labels, and using separate utensils, cutting boards, and cooking surfaces to prevent cross-contamination. You can also play around with different components and recipes to find appropriate replacements for foods that trigger allergies. This way, you can still enjoy a varied and fulfilling diet without sacrificing your health.

Which Techniques Are the Best for Meal Planning and Preparation?

Planning and preparing meals in advance is crucial for keeping a balanced diet, saving time, and lowering stress levels during the hectic workdays. The secret is to schedule specific time each week to organize your meals, make a shopping list, and prep your items ahead of time. Start by selecting recipes for soups, stews, casseroles, and grain bowls that are wholesome, well-balanced, and simple to make in large quantities. After you've decided the recipes you want to try, create a thorough shopping list and stock up on ingredients, making the most of deals and discounts to cut costs. Next, dedicate a few hours to roasting proteins, cooking grains, chopping veggies, and portioning meals into individual containers for convenient grab-and-go. You can organize your weekday dinners more efficiently, cut down on food waste, and make sure you always have wholesome options on hand when hunger hits by setting aside some time in advance for meal prep and planning.

On a tight budget, how can I keep up a healthy diet?

It is feasible to keep a nutritious diet on a tight budget by organizing your meals well, shopping wisely, and preparing your meals strategically. Establish a reasonable budget for groceries and meal preparation at the outset, keeping in mind the dietary requirements and preferences of your family. Look for nutritious and adaptable essentials that are reasonably priced, such as frozen veggies, canned tomatoes, whole grains, beans, lentils, eggs, and reasonably priced meat or poultry pieces. Make dinners centered around these goods, focusing on easy, home-cooked recipes that maximize value and reduce waste. To further minimize costs, shop in bulk whenever you can, take advantage of deals, coupons, and discounts, and think about purchasing store brands or seasonal fruit. Nutrient-dense foods should be prioritized, and you may keep your diet healthy without going over budget if you shop wisely.

Advice on Eating Out While Keeping Up Good Eating Practices

Healthy eating habits might be difficult to maintain when dining out, but you can still choose nutrient-dense choices if you prepare ahead of time and practice mindfulness. Start by checking through the menu ahead of time and selecting items like salads, grilled proteins, and vegetable-based entrees that fit your nutritional tastes and objectives. To avoid excess calories and regulate portion sizes, choose lighter options such as baked, grilled, steamed, or roasted foods. You can also request sauces and dressings on the side. Take note of serving sizes and think about splitting an entrée or getting appetizers instead of a full course. Additionally, to truly appreciate the experience of eating, practice mindful eating by paying attention to your body's signals of hunger and fullness, savoring each bite, and eating deliberately. You may enjoy eating out while still putting your health and wellbeing first by making deliberate decisions and paying attention to your eating habits.

What Effects Does Stress Have on Digestion and General Health?

Stress can have a significant negative effect on digestion and general health, as well as cause a variety of mental and physical symptoms that impair wellbeing. Under stress, the body goes into the "fight or flight" reaction, a condition of hypervigilance that can interfere with regular metabolism and digestion. Many digestive problems, such as gas, bloating, constipation, and irritable bowel syndrome (IBS), can be brought on by prolonged stress. Furthermore, stress can worsen inflammation, impair immunity, and exacerbate a number of chronic illnesses like obesity, diabetes, and heart disease. Prioritizing self-care practices like consistent exercise, enough sleep, relaxing methods like deep breathing or meditation, and asking for help from friends, family, or a healthcare provider can help manage stress and promote general health. Effective stress management can strengthen immunity, facilitate better digestion, and improve your general health and wellbeing.

BREAKFAST RECIPES

Green Smoothie Bowl

Ingredients:

- 1 banana, frozen

- 1 cup spinach leaves

- 1/2 avocado

- 1/2 cup almond milk (or any plant-based milk)

- 1 tablespoon chia seeds

- 1 tablespoon almond butter

- 1 teaspoon honey or maple syrup (optional)

- Fresh fruits, granola, and coconut flakes for topping

Instructions:

1. In a blender, combine the frozen banana, spinach leaves, avocado, almond milk, chia seeds, almond butter, and honey or maple syrup.

2. Blend until smooth and creamy.

3. Pour the smoothie into a bowl.

4. Top with fresh fruits, granola, and coconut flakes.

5. Enjoy immediately!

Nutritional Info (per serving):

- Calories: 350

- Protein: 8g

- Carbohydrates: 40g

- Fat: 18g

- Fiber: 10g

Cook Time: 0 minutes

Prep Time: 10 minutes

Servings: 1

Overnight Chia Pudding

Ingredients:

- 1/4 cup chia seeds

- 1 cup coconut milk (or any plant-based milk)

- 1 tablespoon maple syrup

- 1/2 teaspoon vanilla extract

- Fresh fruits, nuts, and seeds for topping

Instructions:

1. In a bowl, mix the chia seeds, coconut milk, maple syrup, and vanilla extract.

2. Stir well to combine.

3. Cover and refrigerate overnight or for at least 4 hours.

4. In the morning, give it a good stir.

5. Top with fresh fruits, nuts, and seeds before serving.

Nutritional Info (per serving):

- Calories: 250

- Protein: 6g

- Carbohydrates: 22g

- Fat: 16g

- Fiber: 12g

Cook Time: 0 minutes

Prep Time: 5 minutes

Servings: 1

Quinoa Porridge with Berries

Ingredients:

- 1 cup quinoa

- 2 cups water

- 1 cup almond milk

- 1 tablespoon maple syrup

- 1 teaspoon vanilla extract

- 1 cup mixed berries

- Nuts and seeds for topping

Instructions:

1. Rinse the quinoa under cold water.

2. In a saucepan, bring the water to a boil and add the quinoa.

3. Reduce the heat to low, cover, and simmer for 15 minutes.

4. Once the quinoa is cooked, add the almond milk, maple syrup, and vanilla extract.

5. Stir and cook for another 5 minutes until creamy.

6. Serve in bowls and top with mixed berries, nuts, and seeds.

Nutritional Info (per serving):

- Calories: 300

- Protein: 8g

- Carbohydrates: 50g

- Fat: 6g

- Fiber: 6g

Cook Time: 20 minutes

Prep Time: 5 minutes

Servings: 2

Raw Granola with Almond Milk

Ingredients:

- 1 cup rolled oats

- 1/2 cup almonds, chopped

- 1/2 cup sunflower seeds

- 1/4 cup shredded coconut

- 1/4 cup raisins

- 2 tablespoons chia seeds

- 2 tablespoons maple syrup

- 1 teaspoon vanilla extract

- Almond milk for serving

Instructions:

1. In a large bowl, combine the rolled oats, almonds, sunflower seeds, shredded coconut, raisins, and chia seeds.

2. Add the maple syrup and vanilla extract, stirring to coat.

3. Spread the mixture on a baking sheet and let it dry in a dehydrator or oven at the lowest setting until crisp.

4. Serve with almond milk.

Nutritional Info (per serving):

- Calories: 350

- Protein: 10g

- Carbohydrates: 45g

- Fat: 18g

- Fiber: 8g

Cook Time: 0 minutes (if using dehydrator)

Prep Time: 10 minutes

Servings: 4

Avocado Toast with Microgreens

Ingredients:

- 2 slices whole grain bread

- 1 ripe avocado

- 1 tablespoon lemon juice

- Salt and pepper to taste

- Microgreens for topping

Instructions:

1. Toast the whole grain bread slices to your liking.

2. In a bowl, mash the avocado with lemon juice, salt, and pepper.

3. Spread the avocado mixture onto the toasted bread.

4. Top with microgreens and serve immediately.

Nutritional Info (per serving):

- Calories: 250

- Protein: 6g

- Carbohydrates: 28g

- Fat: 16g

- Fiber: 8g

Cook Time: 5 minutes

Prep Time: 5 minutes

Servings: 1

Sprouted Buckwheat Pancakes

Ingredients:

- 1 cup sprouted buckwheat flour
- 1 tablespoon flaxseed meal
- 1 cup almond milk
- 1 tablespoon maple syrup
- 1 teaspoon baking powder
- 1/2 teaspoon vanilla extract
- Coconut oil for cooking

Instructions:

1. In a bowl, mix the sprouted buckwheat flour, flaxseed meal, baking powder, almond milk, maple syrup, and vanilla extract until smooth.
2. Heat a skillet over medium heat and grease with coconut oil.
3. Pour 1/4 cup of batter onto the skillet for each pancake.
4. Cook until bubbles form on the surface, then flip and cook until golden brown.
5. Serve with fresh fruit and maple syrup.

Nutritional Info (per serving):

- Calories: 200
- Protein: 6g
- Carbohydrates: 32g
- Fat: 6g
- Fiber: 5g

Cook Time: 15 minutes

Prep Time: 5 minutes

Servings: 4

Coconut Yogurt Parfait

Ingredients:

- 1 cup coconut yogurt

- 1/2 cup granola

- 1/2 cup fresh berries

- 1 tablespoon chia seeds

- 1 tablespoon honey or maple syrup

Instructions:

1. In a glass or bowl, layer the coconut yogurt, granola, fresh berries, and chia seeds.

2. Drizzle with honey or maple syrup.

3. Repeat the layers until all ingredients are used.

4. Serve immediately or refrigerate until ready to eat.

Nutritional Info (per serving):

- Calories: 300

- Protein: 6g

- Carbohydrates: 40g

- Fat: 12g

- Fiber: 8g

Cook Time: 0 minutes

Prep Time: 5 minutes

Servings: 1

Flaxseed and Berry Smoothie

Ingredients:

- 1 banana

- 1 cup mixed berries (fresh or frozen)

- 1 tablespoon ground flaxseed

- 1 cup almond milk

- 1 tablespoon honey or maple syrup (optional)

- Ice cubes (optional)

Instructions:

1. In a blender, combine the banana, mixed berries, ground flaxseed, almond milk, and honey or maple syrup.

2. Blend until smooth.

3. Add ice cubes if desired and blend again.

4. Pour into a glass and serve immediately.

Nutritional Info (per serving):

- Calories: 250

- Protein: 4g

- Carbohydrates: 45g

- Fat: 6g

- Fiber: 10g

Cook Time: 0 minutes

Prep Time: 5 minutes

Servings: 1

Raw Veggie Wraps with Hummus

Ingredients:

- 4 large collard green leaves

- 1 cup hummus

- 1 carrot, julienned

- 1 cucumber, julienned

- 1 bell pepper, julienned

- 1 avocado, sliced

- 1/4 cup alfalfa sprouts

Instructions:

1. Trim the stems from the collard green leaves.

2. Spread a generous layer of hummus on each leaf.

3. Layer the carrot, cucumber, bell pepper, avocado, and alfalfa sprouts on top of the hummus.

4. Roll the leaves tightly like a burrito.

5. Slice in half and serve.

Nutritional Info (per serving):

- Calories: 200

- Protein: 6g

- Carbohydrates: 25g

- Fat: 10g

- Fiber: 10g

Cook Time: 0 minutes

Prep Time: 10 minutes

Servings: 2

Fermented Coconut Kefir

Ingredients:

- 1 can full-fat coconut milk

- 1 probiotic capsule

Instructions:

1. Pour the coconut milk into a clean glass jar.

2. Open the probiotic capsule and stir the contents into the coconut milk.

3. Cover the jar with a cloth and secure with a rubber band.

4. Let it sit at room temperature for 24-48 hours until it becomes tangy.

5. Refrigerate and use within a week.

Nutritional Info (per serving):

- Calories: 150

- Protein: 2g

- Carbohydrates: 3g

- Fat: 15g

- Fiber: 1g

Cook Time: 0 minutes

Prep Time: 5 minutes

Servings: 4

Herbal Tea with Fresh Mint

Ingredients:

- 2 cups water

- 1 handful fresh mint leaves

- 1 tablespoon honey or to taste (optional)

- Lemon slices for garnish

Instructions:

1. Bring the water to a boil in a small pot.

2. Add the fresh mint leaves and let them steep for 5 minutes.

3. Strain the tea into cups.

4. Sweeten with honey if desired and garnish with lemon slices.

5. Serve hot and enjoy!

Nutritional Info (per serving):

- Calories: 10

- Protein: 0g

- Carbohydrates: 3g

- Fat: 0g

- Fiber: 0g

Cook Time: 5 minutes

Prep Time: 2 minutes

Servings: 2

Raw Nut and Seed Bars

Ingredients:

- 1 cup almonds

- 1/2 cup pumpkin seeds

- 1/2 cup sunflower seeds

- 1/2 cup dried cranberries

- 1/4 cup flaxseeds

- 1/4 cup chia seeds

- 1/2 cup dates, pitted

- 1/4 cup almond butter

- 1/4 cup honey or maple syrup

Instructions:

1. In a food processor, blend the almonds, pumpkin seeds, sunflower seeds, cranberries, flaxseeds, chia seeds, and dates until finely chopped.

2. Add the almond butter and honey, and blend until the mixture sticks together.

3. Press the mixture firmly into a lined baking dish.

4. Refrigerate for at least 2 hours until firm.

5. Cut into bars and store in the fridge.

Nutritional Info (per serving):

- Calories: 250

- Protein: 7g

- Carbohydrates: 24g

- Fat: 15g

- Fiber: 6g

Cook Time: 0 minutes

Prep Time: 15 minutes

Servings: 8

Fresh Fruit Salad with Lemon Dressing

Ingredients:

- 1 cup strawberries, sliced

- 1 cup blueberries

- 1 cup mango, diced

- 1 cup pineapple, diced

- 1 kiwi, sliced

- 2 tablespoons lemon juice

- 1 tablespoon honey or maple syrup

- Fresh mint leaves for garnish

Instructions:

1. In a large bowl, combine the strawberries, blueberries, mango, pineapple, and kiwi.

2. In a small bowl, whisk together the lemon juice and honey.

3. Drizzle the dressing over the fruit and toss gently to combine.

4. Garnish with fresh mint leaves and serve.

Nutritional Info (per serving):

- Calories: 100

- Protein: 1g

- Carbohydrates: 25g

- Fat: 0g

- Fiber: 4g

Cook Time: 0 minutes

Prep Time: 10 minutes

Servings: 4

Raw Almond Butter and Banana Toast

Ingredients:

- 2 slices sprouted grain bread
- 2 tablespoons raw almond butter
- 1 banana, sliced
- 1 teaspoon chia seeds
- A drizzle of honey (optional)

Instructions:

1. Spread the almond butter evenly over the slices of sprouted grain bread.
2. Arrange the banana slices on top of the almond butter.
3. Sprinkle with chia seeds and drizzle with honey if desired.
4. Serve immediately and enjoy!

Nutritional Info (per serving):

- Calories: 300
- Protein: 9g
- Carbohydrates: 35g
- Fat: 15g
- Fiber: 7g

Cook Time: 0 minutes

Prep Time: 5 minutes

Servings: 1

Chia Seed and Coconut Pudding

Ingredients:

- 1/4 cup chia seeds

- 1 cup coconut milk

- 1 tablespoon maple syrup

- 1/2 teaspoon vanilla extract

- Fresh berries for topping

Instructions:

1. In a bowl, mix the chia seeds, coconut milk, maple syrup, and vanilla extract.

2. Stir well to combine.

3. Cover and refrigerate overnight or for at least 4 hours.

4. Give it a good stir in the morning.

5. Top with fresh berries and serve.

Nutritional Info (per serving):

- Calories: 200

- Protein: 4g

- Carbohydrates: 15g

- Fat: 14g

- Fiber: 10g

Cook Time: 0 minutes

Prep Time: 5 minutes

Servings: 2

Green Juice with Spirulina

Ingredients:

- 1 cucumber

- 2 celery stalks

- 1 green apple

- 1 handful spinach

- 1 handful kale

- 1 teaspoon spirulina powder

- Juice of 1 lemon

Instructions:

1. Wash and roughly chop all the produce.

2. Run the cucumber, celery, apple, spinach, and kale through a juicer.

3. Stir in the spirulina powder and lemon juice.

4. Pour into a glass and serve immediately.

Nutritional Info (per serving):

- Calories: 100

- Protein: 3g

- Carbohydrates: 20g

- Fat: 1g

- Fiber: 4g

Cook Time: 0 minutes

Prep Time: 10 minutes

Servings: 2

Raw Apple and Cinnamon Porridge

Ingredients:

- 1 cup rolled oats

- 1 apple, grated

- 1 cup almond milk

- 1 tablespoon maple syrup

- 1 teaspoon cinnamon

- 1/4 cup walnuts, chopped

Instructions:

1. In a bowl, combine the rolled oats, grated apple, almond milk, maple syrup, and cinnamon.

2. Stir well and let it sit for 10 minutes to soften.

3. Top with chopped walnuts and serve.

Nutritional Info (per serving):

- Calories: 250

- Protein: 6g

- Carbohydrates: 40g

- Fat: 9g

- Fiber: 6g

Cook Time: 0 minutes

Prep Time: 10 minutes

Servings: 2

Sprouted Grain Bread with Avocado

Ingredients:

- 2 slices sprouted grain bread

- 1 ripe avocado

- 1 tablespoon lemon juice

- Salt and pepper to taste

- Red pepper flakes (optional)

Instructions:

1. Toast the sprouted grain bread slices to your liking.

2. In a bowl, mash the avocado with lemon juice, salt, and pepper.

3. Spread the avocado mixture onto the toasted bread.

4. Sprinkle with red pepper flakes if desired.

5. Serve immediately.

Nutritional Info (per serving):

- Calories: 250

- Protein: 6g

- Carbohydrates: 28g

- Fat: 16g

- Fiber: 8g

Cook Time: 5 minutes

Prep Time: 5 minutes

Servings: 1

Raw Carrot and Ginger Smoothie

Ingredients:

- 2 carrots, peeled and chopped

- 1 banana

- 1-inch piece of fresh ginger

- 1 cup orange juice

- 1/2 cup almond milk

- Ice cubes (optional)

Instructions:

1. In a blender, combine the carrots, banana, ginger, orange juice, and almond milk.

2. Blend until smooth.

3. Add ice cubes if desired and blend again.

4. Pour into a glass and serve immediately.

Nutritional Info (per serving):

- Calories: 150

- Protein: 2g

- Carbohydrates: 35g

- Fat: 1g

- Fiber: 5g

Cook Time: 0 minutes

Prep Time: 5 minutes

Servings: 1

Herbal Infused Overnight Oats

Ingredients:

- 1 cup rolled oats

- 1 cup herbal tea (chilled)

- 1/2 cup coconut yogurt

- 1 tablespoon honey or maple syrup

- Fresh berries for topping

Instructions:

1. In a bowl, mix the rolled oats, herbal tea, coconut yogurt, and honey.

2. Stir well to combine.

3. Cover and refrigerate overnight.

4. Top with fresh berries in the morning and serve.

Nutritional Info (per serving):

- Calories: 250

- Protein: 6g

- Carbohydrates: 40g

- Fat: 8g

- Fiber: 6g

Cook Time: 0 minutes

Prep Time: 5 minutes

Servings: 2

Raw Vegan Breakfast Burrito

Ingredients:

- 1 large collard green leaf

- 1/2 avocado, sliced

- 1/2 cup shredded carrots

- 1/2 cup shredded cabbage

- 1/4 cup alfalfa sprouts

- 1 tablespoon tahini

- 1 teaspoon lemon juice

- Salt and pepper to taste

Instructions:

1. Trim the stem from the collard green leaf.

2. Spread the tahini over the leaf.

3. Layer the avocado, shredded carrots, shredded cabbage, and alfalfa sprouts on top.

4. Drizzle with lemon juice and season with salt and pepper.

5. Roll the leaf tightly like a burrito.

6. Slice in half and serve.

Nutritional Info (per serving):

- Calories: 150

- Protein: 4g

- Carbohydrates: 15g

- Fat: 10g

- Fiber

CONITUE

ChatGPT

: 6g

Cook Time: 0 minutes

Prep Time: 10 minutes

Servings: 1

Hemp Seed and Blueberry Smoothie

Ingredients:

- 1 banana

- 1 cup blueberries (fresh or frozen)

- 1 tablespoon hemp seeds

- 1 cup almond milk

- 1 tablespoon honey or maple syrup (optional)

- Ice cubes (optional)

Instructions:

1. In a blender, combine the banana, blueberries, hemp seeds, almond milk, and honey or maple syrup.

2. Blend until smooth.

3. Add ice cubes if desired and blend again.

4. Pour into a glass and serve immediately.

Nutritional Info (per serving):

- Calories: 250

- Protein: 6g

- Carbohydrates: 45g

- Fat: 8g

- Fiber: 7g

Cook Time: 0 minutes

Prep Time: 5 minutes

Servings: 1

Raw Cashew and Berry Parfait

Ingredients:

- 1 cup cashews, soaked overnight

- 1/2 cup water

- 1 tablespoon maple syrup

- 1 teaspoon vanilla extract

- 1 cup mixed berries

- 1/4 cup granola

Instructions:

1. In a blender, combine the soaked cashews, water, maple syrup, and vanilla extract.

2. Blend until smooth and creamy.

3. In a glass or bowl, layer the cashew cream, mixed berries, and granola.

4. Repeat the layers until all ingredients are used.

5. Serve immediately or refrigerate until ready to eat.

Nutritional Info (per serving):

- Calories: 300

- Protein: 8g

- Carbohydrates: 30g

- Fat: 18g

- Fiber: 4g

Cook Time: 0 minutes

Prep Time: 10 minutes

Servings: 2

Fermented Vegetable and Grain Bowl

Ingredients:

- 1 cup cooked quinoa or brown rice

- 1/2 cup fermented vegetables (such as sauerkraut or kimchi)

- 1/2 avocado, sliced

- 1/2 cup shredded carrots

- 1/2 cup sliced cucumber

- 1 tablespoon sesame seeds

- 1 tablespoon tamari or soy sauce

- 1 teaspoon sesame oil

Instructions:

1. In a bowl, combine the cooked quinoa or brown rice, fermented vegetables, avocado, shredded carrots, and cucumber.

2. Drizzle with tamari or soy sauce and sesame oil.

3. Sprinkle with sesame seeds.

4. Toss gently to combine and serve.

Nutritional Info (per serving):

- Calories: 300

- Protein: 8g

- Carbohydrates: 35g

- Fat: 14g

- Fiber: 8g

Cook Time: 0 minutes

Prep Time: 10 minutes

Servings: 2

Raw Cacao and Banana Smoothie

Ingredients:

- 1 banana

- 1 tablespoon raw cacao powder

- 1 cup almond milk

- 1 tablespoon almond butter

- 1 teaspoon honey or maple syrup (optional)

- Ice cubes (optional)

Instructions:

1. In a blender, combine the banana, raw cacao powder, almond milk, almond butter, and honey or maple syrup.

2. Blend until smooth.

3. Add ice cubes if desired and blend again.

4. Pour into a glass and serve immediately.

Nutritional Info (per serving):

- Calories: 200

- Protein: 5g

- Carbohydrates: 30g

- Fat: 9g

- Fiber: 5g

Cook Time: 0 minutes

Prep Time: 5 minutes

Servings: 1

Almond and Date Energy Bites

Ingredients:

- 1 cup almonds

- 1 cup pitted dates

- 1/4 cup shredded coconut

- 1 tablespoon chia seeds

- 1 tablespoon coconut oil

- 1 teaspoon vanilla extract

Instructions:

1. In a food processor, blend the almonds and dates until finely chopped.

2. Add the shredded coconut, chia seeds, coconut oil, and vanilla extract.

3. Blend until the mixture comes together.

4. Roll into small balls and place on a lined baking sheet.

5. Refrigerate for at least 1 hour until firm.

6. Store in the fridge.

Nutritional Info (per serving):

- Calories: 100

- Protein: 2g

- Carbohydrates: 15g

- Fat: 5g

- Fiber: 3g

Cook Time: 0 minutes

Prep Time: 10 minutes

Servings: 12

Raw Broccoli and Spinach Smoothie

Ingredients:

- 1 cup broccoli florets

- 1 cup spinach leaves

- 1 banana

- 1 apple, cored and chopped

- 1 cup coconut water

- 1 tablespoon lemon juice

- Ice cubes (optional)

Instructions:

1. In a blender, combine the broccoli, spinach, banana, apple, coconut water, and lemon juice.

2. Blend until smooth.

3. Add ice cubes if desired and blend again.

4. Pour into a glass and serve immediately.

Nutritional Info (per serving):

- Calories: 150

- Protein: 3g

- Carbohydrates: 35g

- Fat: 1g

- Fiber: 7g

Cook Time: 0 minutes

Prep Time: 5 minutes

Servings: 1

Raw Pumpkin Seed Granola

Ingredients:

- 1 cup rolled oats

- 1/2 cup pumpkin seeds

- 1/4 cup sunflower seeds

- 1/4 cup shredded coconut

- 1/4 cup dried cranberries

- 2 tablespoons chia seeds

- 2 tablespoons maple syrup

- 1 teaspoon vanilla extract

Instructions:

1. In a large bowl, combine the rolled oats, pumpkin seeds, sunflower seeds, shredded coconut, dried cranberries, and chia seeds.

2. Add the maple syrup and vanilla extract, stirring to coat.

3. Spread the mixture on a baking sheet and let it dry in a dehydrator or oven at the lowest setting until crisp.

4. Store in an airtight container.

Nutritional Info (per serving):

- Calories: 200

- Protein: 6g

- Carbohydrates: 30g

- Fat: 8g

- Fiber: 5g

Cook Time: 0 minutes (if using dehydrator)

Prep Time: 10 minutes

Servings: 6

Fresh Coconut Water and Fruit Bowl

Ingredients:

- 1 young coconut

- 1 cup mixed tropical fruits (such as pineapple, mango, and kiwi)

- 1 tablespoon fresh lime juice

- Fresh mint leaves for garnish

Instructions:

1. Carefully open the young coconut and pour the coconut water into a bowl.

2. Scoop out the coconut meat and add it to the bowl.

3. Add the mixed tropical fruits and lime juice.

4. Garnish with fresh mint leaves.

5. Serve immediately.

Nutritional Info (per serving):

- Calories: 150

- Protein: 2g

- Carbohydrates: 30g

- Fat: 3g

- Fiber: 4g

Cook Time: 0 minutes

Prep Time: 10 minutes

Servings: 2

Raw Sunflower Seed Spread on Sprouted Bread

Ingredients:

- 1 cup sunflower seeds, soaked overnight

- 1/4 cup water

- 1 tablespoon lemon juice

- 1 tablespoon tahini

- 1 garlic clove

- Salt and pepper to taste

- 2 slices sprouted grain bread

Instructions:

1. In a food processor, blend the soaked sunflower seeds, water, lemon juice, tahini, garlic, salt, and pepper until smooth.

2. Spread the sunflower seed mixture onto the sprouted grain bread slices.

3. Serve immediately and enjoy.

Nutritional Info (per serving):

- Calories: 250

- Protein: 8g

- Carbohydrates: 22g

- Fat: 15g

- Fiber: 6g

Cook Time: 0 minutes

Prep Time: 10 minutes

Servings: 2

LUNCH RECIPES

Raw Zucchini Noodles with Pesto

Ingredients:

- 4 medium zucchinis

- 1 cup fresh basil leaves

- 1/2 cup raw walnuts

- 2 cloves garlic, minced

- 1/4 cup nutritional yeast

- 1/4 cup extra-virgin olive oil

- Salt and pepper, to taste

Instructions:

1. Using a spiralizer, create zucchini noodles and set aside in a large bowl.

2. In a food processor, combine basil, walnuts, garlic, and nutritional yeast. Pulse until finely chopped.

3. Slowly add olive oil while continuing to pulse until the mixture becomes a smooth pesto.

4. Season with salt and pepper to taste.

5. Toss the zucchini noodles with the pesto until evenly coated.

6. Serve immediately or refrigerate for up to two days.

Nutritional Info (per serving):

- Calories: 250

- Protein: 7g

- Carbohydrates: 10g

- Fat: 22g

- Fiber: 4g

Cook Time: None **Prep Time:** 15 minutes *Servings:* 4

Sprouted Lentil Salad with Lemon Tahini Dressing

Ingredients:

- 1 cup sprouted lentils

- 1 red bell pepper, diced

- 1 cucumber, diced

- 1/4 cup chopped fresh parsley

- 1/4 cup lemon juice

- 2 tablespoons tahini

- 2 tablespoons extra-virgin olive oil

- 1 clove garlic, minced

- Salt and pepper, to taste

Instructions:

1. In a large bowl, combine sprouted lentils, bell pepper, cucumber, and parsley.

2. In a small bowl, whisk together lemon juice, tahini, olive oil, garlic, salt, and pepper.

3. Pour the dressing over the lentil mixture and toss to combine.

4. Serve immediately or refrigerate for up to three days.

Nutritional Info (per serving):

- Calories: 230

- Protein: 9g

- Carbohydrates: 21g

- Fat: 13g

- Fiber: 8g

Cook Time: None (assuming lentils are pre-sprouted) **Prep Time:** 15 minutes *Servings:* 4

Raw Veggie Sushi Rolls

Ingredients:

- 4 nori sheets

- 2 cups cauliflower rice

- 1 avocado, thinly sliced

- 1 cucumber, julienned

- 1 carrot, julienned

- 1/2 red bell pepper, julienned

- Tamari or coconut aminos, for dipping (optional)

Instructions:

1. Place a nori sheet on a flat surface.

2. Spread a thin layer of cauliflower rice over the nori, leaving about an inch of space at the top.

3. Arrange avocado, cucumber, carrot, and bell pepper in a line across the rice.

4. Starting from the bottom, tightly roll the nori sheet into a cylinder, using a bit of water to seal the edge.

5. Repeat with remaining nori sheets and filling.

6. Slice the rolls into bite-sized pieces.

7. Serve with tamari or coconut aminos for dipping, if desired.

Nutritional Info (per serving):

- Calories: 180

- Protein: 5g

- Carbohydrates: 24g

- Fat: 8g

- Fiber: 7g

Cook Time: None **Prep Time:** 20 minutes *Servings:* 4

Fermented Vegetable and Quinoa Bowl

Ingredients:

- 1 cup cooked quinoa

- 1 cup mixed fermented vegetables (such as sauerkraut, kimchi, or pickles)

- 1/2 cup cooked black beans

- 1/2 avocado, diced

- 1 tablespoon hemp seeds

- 1 tablespoon olive oil

- 1 tablespoon lemon juice

- Salt and pepper, to taste

Instructions:

1. In a bowl, combine quinoa, fermented vegetables, black beans, avocado, and hemp seeds.

2. Drizzle with olive oil and lemon juice.

3. Season with salt and pepper to taste.

4. Toss gently to combine.

5. Serve immediately.

Nutritional Info (per serving):

- Calories: 380

- Protein: 12g

- Carbohydrates: 46g

- Fat: 18g

- Fiber: 11g

Cook Time: 15 minutes (for quinoa) **Prep Time:** 10 minutes *Servings:* 2

Avocado and Sprout Wraps

Ingredients:

- 4 large collard green leaves

- 1 avocado, mashed

- 1 cup mixed sprouts (such as alfalfa, broccoli, or radish)

- 1/2 red bell pepper, thinly sliced

- 1/2 cucumber, thinly sliced

- 1/4 cup shredded carrots

- 1/4 cup hummus

- Salt and pepper, to taste

Instructions:

1. Lay a collard green leaf flat on a cutting board.

2. Spread a quarter of the mashed avocado down the center of the leaf.

3. Top with a quarter of the sprouts, bell pepper, cucumber, and carrots.

4. Season with salt and pepper.

5. Roll the leaf tightly, tucking in the sides as you go.

6. Repeat with remaining ingredients.

7. Slice each wrap in half.

8. Serve immediately.

Nutritional Info (per serving):

- Calories: 180

- Protein: 6g

- Carbohydrates: 21g

- Fat: 10g

- Fiber: 10g

Cook Time: None **Prep Time:** 15 minutes *Servings:* 4

Raw Cauliflower Rice with Herbs

Ingredients:

- 1 head cauliflower, chopped into florets
- 1/4 cup fresh parsley, chopped
- 2 tablespoons fresh mint, chopped
- 2 tablespoons fresh dill, chopped
- 2 tablespoons lemon juice
- 2 tablespoons extra-virgin olive oil
- Salt and pepper, to taste

Instructions:

1. Place cauliflower florets in a food processor and pulse until they resemble rice-like grains.
2. Transfer the cauliflower rice to a large bowl.
3. Add chopped parsley, mint, and dill to the cauliflower rice.
4. Drizzle with lemon juice and olive oil.
5. Season with salt and pepper to taste.
6. Toss until well combined.
7. Serve immediately or refrigerate until ready to serve.

Nutritional Info (per serving):

- Calories: 80
- Protein: 3g
- Carbohydrates: 6g

- Fat: 6g

- Fiber: 3g

Cook Time: None **Prep Time:** 10 minutes *Servings:* 4

Fresh Tomato and Basil Gazpacho

Ingredients:

- 6 large tomatoes, chopped

- 1 cucumber, peeled and chopped

- 1 red bell pepper, chopped

- 1/4 red onion, chopped

- 2 cloves garlic, minced

- 1/4 cup fresh basil leaves

- 2 tablespoons red wine vinegar

- 2 tablespoons extra-virgin olive oil

- Salt and pepper, to taste

Instructions:

1. In a blender, combine chopped tomatoes, cucumber, bell pepper, onion, garlic, and basil leaves.

2. Blend until smooth.

3. Stir in red wine vinegar and olive oil.

4. Season with salt and pepper to taste.

5. Chill in the refrigerator for at least 1 hour before serving.

6. Serve cold, garnished with additional basil leaves if desired.

Nutritional Info (per serving):

- Calories: 90

- Protein: 2g

- Carbohydrates: 10g

- Fat: 6g

- Fiber: 3g

Cook Time: None **Prep Time:** 15 minutes *Servings:* 4

Raw Walnut and Sun-Dried Tomato Tacos

Ingredients:

- 8 large lettuce leaves (such as romaine or butter lettuce)

- 1 cup raw walnuts

- 1/2 cup sun-dried tomatoes (not in oil)

- 1 tablespoon tamari or soy sauce

- 1 teaspoon chili powder

- 1 teaspoon ground cumin

- 1 avocado, sliced

- 1/4 cup diced red onion

- 1/4 cup chopped fresh cilantro

- Lime wedges, for serving

Instructions:

1. In a food processor, pulse walnuts and sun-dried tomatoes until finely chopped.

2. Add tamari, chili powder, and cumin. Pulse until well combined.

3. Spoon walnut mixture onto lettuce leaves.

4. Top with avocado slices, diced red onion, and chopped cilantro.

5. Squeeze fresh lime juice over the tacos before serving.

Nutritional Info (per serving):

- Calories: 280

- Protein: 7g

- Carbohydrates: 12g

- Fat: 24g

- Fiber: 7g

Cook Time: None **Prep Time:** 15 minutes *Servings:* 4

Sprouted Chickpea Salad with Fresh Herbs

Ingredients:

- 2 cups sprouted chickpeas

- 1 cup cherry tomatoes, halved

- 1/2 cucumber, diced

- 1/4 cup chopped fresh parsley

- 1/4 cup chopped fresh mint

- 1/4 cup chopped fresh cilantro

- 2 tablespoons lemon juice

- 2 tablespoons extra-virgin olive oil

- Salt and pepper, to taste

Instructions:

1. In a large bowl, combine sprouted chickpeas, cherry tomatoes, cucumber, parsley, mint, and cilantro.

2. Drizzle with lemon juice and olive oil.

3. Season with salt and pepper to taste.

4. Toss gently until all ingredients are evenly coated.

5. Serve immediately or refrigerate until ready to serve.

Nutritional Info (per serving):

- Calories: 180

- Protein: 7g

- Carbohydrates: 19g

- Fat: 9g

- Fiber: 6g

Cook Time: None (assuming chickpeas are pre-sprouted) **Prep Time:** 10 minutes *Servings:* 4

Raw Beet and Carrot Slaw

Ingredients:

- 2 medium beets, peeled and grated
- 2 medium carrots, peeled and grated
- 1/4 cup chopped fresh parsley
- 1/4 cup chopped fresh cilantro
- 2 tablespoons lemon juice
- 2 tablespoons extra-virgin olive oil
- Salt and pepper, to taste

Instructions:

1. In a large bowl, combine grated beets, grated carrots, parsley, and cilantro.
2. Drizzle with lemon juice and olive oil.
3. Season with salt and pepper to taste.
4. Toss until well combined.
5. Serve immediately or refrigerate until ready to serve.

Nutritional Info (per serving):

- Calories: 120
- Protein: 2g
- Carbohydrates: 11g
- Fat: 8g
- Fiber: 3g

Cook Time: None **Prep Time:** 10 minutes *Servings:* 4

Raw Veggie Wrap with Hummus

Ingredients:

- 4 large collard green leaves
- 1/2 cup hummus
- 1 cucumber, julienned
- 1 carrot, julienned
- 1/2 red bell pepper, julienned
- 1/4 cup alfalfa sprouts
- 1/4 cup shredded purple cabbage
- 1/4 cup shredded carrots

Instructions:

1. Lay a collard green leaf flat on a cutting board.
2. Spread a layer of hummus evenly over the leaf.
3. Layer cucumber, carrot, bell pepper, alfalfa sprouts, purple cabbage, and shredded carrots on top of the hummus.
4. Roll the leaf tightly, tucking in the sides as you go.
5. Repeat with remaining ingredients.
6. Slice each wrap in half.
7. Serve immediately.

Nutritional Info (per serving):

- Calories: 120

- Protein: 5g

- Carbohydrates: 18g

- Fat: 4g

- Fiber: 8g

Cook Time: None **Prep Time:** 15 minutes *Servings:* 4

Cabbage and Apple Slaw with Ginger Dressing

Ingredients:

- 1/2 head green cabbage, thinly sliced

- 1 apple, julienned

- 1/4 cup chopped fresh cilantro

- 2 tablespoons apple cider vinegar

- 1 tablespoon maple syrup

- 1 tablespoon grated fresh ginger

- 1 tablespoon sesame oil

- Salt and pepper, to taste

- Sesame seeds, for garnish

Instructions:

1. In a large bowl, combine sliced cabbage, julienned apple, and chopped cilantro.

2. In a small bowl, whisk together apple cider vinegar, maple syrup, grated ginger, sesame oil, salt, and pepper.

3. Pour the dressing over the cabbage mixture and toss until well coated.

4. Sprinkle with sesame seeds before serving.

Nutritional Info (per serving):

- Calories: 90

- Protein: 1g

- Carbohydrates: 14g

- Fat: 4g

- Fiber: 3g

Cook Time: None **Prep Time:** 10 minutes *Servings:* 4

Raw Spinach and Strawberry Salad

Ingredients:

- 6 cups baby spinach leaves

- 2 cups sliced strawberries

- 1/4 cup sliced almonds

- 1/4 cup crumbled feta cheese (optional)

- 2 tablespoons balsamic vinegar

- 1 tablespoon extra-virgin olive oil

- 1 teaspoon honey

- Salt and pepper, to taste

Instructions:

1. In a large bowl, combine baby spinach, sliced strawberries, sliced almonds, and crumbled feta cheese.

2. In a small bowl, whisk together balsamic vinegar, olive oil, honey, salt, and pepper.

3. Drizzle the dressing over the salad and toss gently to combine.

4. Serve immediately.

Nutritional Info (per serving):

- Calories: 150

- Protein: 4g

- Carbohydrates: 14g

- Fat: 9g

- Fiber: 5g

Cook Time: None **Prep Time:** 10 minutes *Servings:* 4

Fermented Cabbage and Apple Salad

Ingredients:

- 4 cups shredded green cabbage

- 1 apple, thinly sliced

- 2 tablespoons apple cider vinegar

- 1 teaspoon sea salt

- 1 teaspoon caraway seeds (optional)

- 1/4 cup water (if needed)

Instructions:

1. In a large bowl, combine shredded cabbage, sliced apple, apple cider vinegar, sea salt, and caraway seeds (if using).

2. Massage the cabbage and apple mixture with clean hands for about 5 minutes, or until they start to release their juices.

3. If the mixture seems dry, add water, 1 tablespoon at a time, until the cabbage and apple are submerged.

4. Transfer the mixture to a clean glass jar, pressing it down firmly to remove any air bubbles and ensure it is submerged in liquid.

5. Cover the jar loosely with a lid or a clean cloth secured with a rubber band.

6. Allow the salad to ferment at room temperature for 3 to 7 days, depending on desired level of fermentation.

7. Once fermented to your liking, transfer the jar to the refrigerator to slow down the fermentation process.

8. Serve chilled as a side dish or topping for sandwiches and salads.

Nutritional Info (per serving):

- Calories: 30

- Protein: 1g

- Carbohydrates: 7g

- Fat: 0g

- Fiber: 3g

Cook Time: None *Prep Time:* 15 minutes (plus fermentation time) *Servings:* 4

Raw Vegan Pad Thai

Ingredients:

- 2 medium zucchinis, spiralized

- 1 large carrot, julienned

- 1 red bell pepper, thinly sliced

- 1/2 cup shredded purple cabbage

- 1/4 cup chopped fresh cilantro

- 1/4 cup chopped peanuts

- Lime wedges, for serving

- Optional: sliced green onions, bean sprouts

Sauce:

- 1/4 cup almond butter

- 2 tablespoons tamari or soy sauce

- 2 tablespoons lime juice

- 1 tablespoon maple syrup

- 1 clove garlic, minced

- 1 teaspoon grated ginger

- 1/4 teaspoon red pepper flakes

Instructions:

1. In a large bowl, combine spiralized zucchini, julienned carrot, sliced bell pepper, shredded cabbage, and chopped cilantro.

2. In a small bowl, whisk together almond butter, tamari, lime juice, maple syrup, garlic, ginger, and red pepper flakes to make the sauce.

3. Pour the sauce over the vegetable mixture and toss until well coated.

4. Divide the pad Thai among plates and top with chopped peanuts.

5. Serve with lime wedges and optional toppings like sliced green onions and bean sprouts.

Nutritional Info (per serving):

- Calories: 280

- Protein: 9g

- Carbohydrates: 20g

- Fat: 20g

- Fiber: 6g

Cook Time: None **Prep Time:** 20 minutes *Servings:* 4

Fresh Cucumber and Avocado Salad

Ingredients:

- 2 large cucumbers, thinly sliced

- 1 avocado, diced

- 1/4 cup chopped fresh dill

- 2 tablespoons lemon juice

- 1 tablespoon extra-virgin olive oil

- Salt and pepper, to taste

Instructions:

1. In a large bowl, combine sliced cucumbers, diced avocado, and chopped dill.

2. Drizzle with lemon juice and olive oil.

3. Season with salt and pepper to taste.

4. Toss gently until well combined.

5. Serve immediately.

Nutritional Info (per serving):

- Calories: 120

- Protein: 2g

- Carbohydrates: 10g

- Fat: 9g

- Fiber: 4g

Cook Time: None **Prep Time:** 10 minutes *Servings:* 4

Raw Carrot and Coconut Soup

Ingredients:

- 4 large carrots, chopped

- 1 can (13.5 oz) full-fat coconut milk

- 2 cups vegetable broth

- 1 tablespoon fresh ginger, grated

- 1 clove garlic, minced

- 1 tablespoon lime juice

- Salt and pepper, to taste

- Optional toppings: chopped cilantro, coconut flakes, lime wedges

Instructions:

1. In a blender, combine chopped carrots, coconut milk, vegetable broth, ginger, garlic, lime juice, salt, and pepper.

2. Blend until smooth and creamy.

3. If the soup is too thick, add more vegetable broth or water to reach the desired consistency.

4. Pour the soup into bowls and garnish with chopped cilantro, coconut flakes, and lime wedges, if desired.

5. Serve chilled or at room temperature.

Nutritional Info (per serving):

- Calories: 250

- Protein: 3g

- Carbohydrates: 17g

- Fat: 21g

- Fiber: 4g

Cook Time: None **Prep Time:** 15 minutes *Servings:* 4

Sprouted Grain and Veggie Bowl

Ingredients:

- 2 cups cooked sprouted grains (such as quinoa, brown rice, or barley)

- 1 cup mixed vegetables (such as bell peppers, zucchini, and broccoli), diced

- 1/4 cup chopped fresh parsley

- 2 tablespoons lemon juice

- 2 tablespoons extra-virgin olive oil

- Salt and pepper, to taste

- Optional toppings: avocado slices, hemp seeds

Instructions:

1. In a large bowl, combine cooked sprouted grains, diced vegetables, and chopped parsley.

2. Drizzle with lemon juice and olive oil.

3. Season with salt and pepper to taste.

4. Toss gently until well combined.

5. Serve warm or at room temperature, topped with avocado slices and hemp seeds if desired.

Nutritional Info (per serving):

- Calories: 280

- Protein: 8g

- Carbohydrates: 40g

- Fat: 10g

- Fiber: 8g

Cook Time: Varies (depends on the grains) **Prep Time:** 15 minutes *Servings:* 4

Raw Sweet Potato and Kale Salad

Ingredients:

- 2 medium sweet potatoes, peeled and grated
- 4 cups chopped kale leaves
- 1/4 cup dried cranberries
- 1/4 cup chopped pecans
- 2 tablespoons apple cider vinegar
- 1 tablespoon maple syrup
- 1 tablespoon extra-virgin olive oil
- Salt and pepper, to taste

Instructions:

1. In a large bowl, combine grated sweet potatoes, chopped kale, dried cranberries, and chopped pecans.
2. In a small bowl, whisk together apple cider vinegar, maple syrup, olive oil, salt, and pepper.
3. Pour the dressing over the salad and toss until well coated.
4. Serve immediately or refrigerate until ready to serve.

Nutritional Info (per serving):

- Calories: 220
- Protein: 4g
- Carbohydrates: 35g
- Fat: 8g

- Fiber: 6g

Cook Time: None **Prep Time:** 15 minutes *Servings:* 4

Fermented Kimchi and Veggie Wrap

Ingredients:

- 4 large collard green leaves
- 1/2 cup fermented kimchi
- 1/2 cucumber, julienned
- 1 carrot, julienned
- 1/2 red bell pepper, julienned
- 1/4 cup chopped fresh cilantro
- 1/4 cup hummus
- Optional: sliced avocado, sesame seeds

Instructions:

1. Lay a collard green leaf flat on a cutting board.
2. Spread a thin layer of hummus over the leaf.
3. Layer kimchi, cucumber, carrot, bell pepper, and cilantro on top of the hummus.
4. Add sliced avocado and sprinkle with sesame seeds, if desired.
5. Roll the leaf tightly, tucking in the sides as you go.
6. Repeat with remaining ingredients.
7. Slice each wrap in half.

8. Serve immediately.

Nutritional Info (per serving):

- Calories: 120

- Protein: 4g

- Carbohydrates: 18g

- Fat: 4g

- Fiber: 8g

Cook Time: None **Prep Time:** 15 minutes *Servings:*

Raw Asparagus and Avocado Salad

Ingredients:

- 1 bunch asparagus, ends trimmed and thinly sliced

- 1 avocado, diced

- 1/4 cup chopped fresh parsley

- 2 tablespoons lemon juice

- 1 tablespoon extra-virgin olive oil

- Salt and pepper, to taste

- Optional: hemp seeds, pine nuts

Instructions:

1. In a large bowl, combine sliced asparagus, diced avocado, and chopped parsley.

2. Drizzle with lemon juice and olive oil.

3. Season with salt and pepper to taste.

4. Toss gently until well combined.

5. Sprinkle with hemp seeds or pine nuts, if desired.

6. Serve immediately.

Nutritional Info (per serving):

- Calories: 180

- Protein: 5g

- Carbohydrates: 12g

- Fat: 14g

- Fiber: 7g

Cook Time: None **Prep Time:** 10 minutes *Servings:* 4

Sprouted Black Bean and Corn Salad

Ingredients:

- 2 cups cooked sprouted black beans

- 1 cup corn kernels (fresh or thawed if frozen)

- 1 red bell pepper, diced

- 1/4 cup chopped red onion

- 1/4 cup chopped fresh cilantro

- 2 tablespoons lime juice

- 1 tablespoon extra-virgin olive oil

- 1 teaspoon ground cumin

- Salt and pepper, to taste

- Optional: diced avocado, jalapeño slices

Instructions:

1. In a large bowl, combine sprouted black beans, corn kernels, diced bell pepper, red onion, and cilantro.

2. In a small bowl, whisk together lime juice, olive oil, cumin, salt, and pepper.

3. Pour the dressing over the bean mixture and toss until well coated.

4. Serve chilled or at room temperature.

5. Top with diced avocado and jalapeño slices, if desired.

Nutritional Info (per serving):

- Calories: 210

- Protein: 9g

- Carbohydrates: 35g

- Fat: 5g

- Fiber: 10g

Cook Time: None (assuming beans are pre-sprouted) **Prep Time:** 15 minutes *Servings:* 4

Raw Broccoli and Cashew Stir-Fry

Ingredients:

- 4 cups chopped broccoli florets

- 1/2 cup cashews

- 1 red bell pepper, thinly sliced

- 1/2 cup sliced mushrooms

- 1/4 cup chopped green onions

- 2 tablespoons tamari or soy sauce

- 2 tablespoons sesame oil

- 1 tablespoon rice vinegar

- 1 tablespoon maple syrup

- 1 teaspoon grated ginger

- 1 clove garlic, minced

- Optional: cooked quinoa or brown rice

Instructions:

1. In a large bowl, combine chopped broccoli, cashews, sliced bell pepper, mushrooms, and green onions.

2. In a small bowl, whisk together tamari, sesame oil, rice vinegar, maple syrup, ginger, and garlic.

3. Pour the sauce over the broccoli mixture and toss until well coated.

4. Serve as is or over cooked quinoa or brown rice.

Nutritional Info (per serving, without quinoa or rice):

- Calories: 250

- Protein: 9g

- Carbohydrates: 18g

- Fat: 18g

- Fiber: 5g

Cook Time: None **Prep Time:** 15 minutes *Servings:* 4

Fresh Garden Salad with Lemon Vinaigrette

Ingredients:

- 6 cups mixed salad greens (such as lettuce, spinach, arugula)

- 1 cup cherry tomatoes, halved

- 1/2 cucumber, sliced

- 1/4 cup sliced red onion

- 1/4 cup sliced radishes

- 1/4 cup sliced black olives

- Lemon Vinaigrette:

    - 1/4 cup fresh lemon juice

    - 1/4 cup extra-virgin olive oil

    - 1 teaspoon Dijon mustard

    - 1 teaspoon maple syrup

    - Salt and pepper, to taste

Instructions:

1. In a large bowl, combine mixed salad greens, cherry tomatoes, cucumber, red onion, radishes, and black olives.

2. In a small bowl, whisk together lemon juice, olive oil, Dijon mustard, maple syrup, salt, and pepper to make the vinaigrette.

3. Pour the vinaigrette over the salad and toss gently to coat.

4. Serve immediately.

Nutritional Info (per serving):

- Calories: 150

- Protein: 2g

- Carbohydrates: 9g

- Fat: 12g

- Fiber: 3g

Cook Time: None **Prep Time:** 15 minutes *Servings:* 4

Raw Red Pepper and Walnut Dip with Veggies

Ingredients:

- 2 red bell peppers, roasted and peeled

- 1 cup raw walnuts

- 1 clove garlic

- 2 tablespoons lemon juice

- 2 tablespoons extra-virgin olive oil

- Salt and pepper, to taste

- Assorted raw vegetables for dipping (carrots, cucumbers, bell peppers, etc.)

Instructions:

1. In a food processor, combine roasted red peppers, walnuts, garlic, lemon juice, olive oil, salt, and pepper.

2. Blend until smooth and creamy.

3. Transfer the dip to a serving bowl.

4. Serve with assorted raw vegetables for dipping.

Nutritional Info (per serving):

- Calories: 150

- Protein: 3g

- Carbohydrates: 6g

- Fat: 14g

- Fiber: 2g

Cook Time: 15 minutes (for roasting peppers) **Prep Time:** 10 minutes *Servings:* 4

Sprouted Mung Bean Salad

Ingredients:

- 1 cup sprouted mung beans

- 1 cucumber, diced

- 1 tomato, diced

- 1/4 cup chopped red onion

- 1/4 cup chopped fresh cilantro

- 2 tablespoons lemon juice

- 2 tablespoons extra-virgin olive oil

- Salt and pepper, to taste

Instructions:

1. In a large bowl, combine sprouted mung beans, diced cucumber, diced tomato, chopped red onion, and chopped cilantro.

2. Drizzle with lemon juice and olive oil.

3. Season with salt and pepper to taste.

4. Toss gently until well combined.

5. Serve chilled or at room temperature.

Nutritional Info (per serving):

- Calories: 160

- Protein: 6g

- Carbohydrates: 18g

- Fat: 8g

- Fiber: 5g

Cook Time: None (assuming mung beans are pre-sprouted) **Prep Time:** 15 minutes *Servings:* 4

Raw Cucumber and Dill Soup

Ingredients:

- 2 large cucumbers, peeled and chopped

- 1/2 cup raw cashews, soaked for 2 hours and drained

- 1/4 cup chopped fresh dill

- 2 tablespoons lemon juice

- 1 clove garlic

- 2 cups water

- Salt and pepper, to taste

Instructions:

1. In a blender, combine chopped cucumbers, soaked cashews, chopped dill, lemon juice, garlic, and water.

2. Blend until smooth and creamy.

3. Season with salt and pepper to taste.

4. Chill in the refrigerator for at least 1 hour before serving.

5. Serve cold, garnished with additional dill if desired.

Nutritional Info (per serving):

- Calories: 180

- Protein: 6g

- Carbohydrates: 14g

- Fat: 12g

- Fiber: 3g

Cook Time: None **Prep Time:** 10 minutes (plus soaking time for cashews) *Servings:* 4

Fermented Beet and Carrot Salad

Ingredients:

- 2 beets, peeled and grated

- 2 carrots, peeled and grated

- 1/4 cup chopped fresh dill

- 2 tablespoons apple cider vinegar

- 1 tablespoon maple syrup

- 1 teaspoon sea salt

- 1/2 teaspoon caraway seeds

- 1/4 cup water (if needed)

Instructions:

1. In a large bowl, combine grated beets, grated carrots, chopped dill, apple cider vinegar, maple syrup, sea salt, and caraway seeds.

2. Massage the vegetables with clean hands for about 5 minutes, or until they start to release their juices.

3. If the mixture seems dry, add water, 1 tablespoon at a time, until the vegetables are submerged.

4. Transfer the mixture to a clean glass jar, pressing it down firmly to remove any air bubbles and ensure it is submerged in liquid.

5. Cover the jar loosely with a lid or a clean cloth secured with a rubber band.

6. Allow the salad to ferment at room temperature for 3 to 7 days, depending on desired level of fermentation.

7. Once fermented to your liking, transfer the jar to the refrigerator to slow down the fermentation process.

8. Serve chilled as a side dish or topping for salads and sandwiches.

Nutritional Info (per serving):

- Calories: 70

- Protein: 2g

- Carbohydrates: 16g

- Fat: 1g

- Fiber: 4g

Raw Collard Green Wraps with Almond Butter

Ingredients:

- 4 large collard green leaves
- 1/2 cup almond butter
- 1 banana, thinly sliced
- 1/4 cup chopped nuts (such as almonds, walnuts, or pecans)
- 1/4 cup shredded coconut
- 1/4 cup raisins or dried cranberries
- Optional: drizzle of honey or maple syrup

Instructions:

1. Lay a collard green leaf flat on a cutting board.
2. Spread a layer of almond butter evenly over the leaf.
3. Arrange sliced banana, chopped nuts, shredded coconut, and raisins or dried cranberries on top of the almond butter.
4. Drizzle with honey or maple syrup, if desired.
5. Roll the leaf tightly, tucking in the sides as you go.
6. Repeat with remaining ingredients.
7. Slice each wrap in half.
8. Serve immediately.

Nutritional Info (per serving):

- Calories: 380

- Protein: 9g

- Carbohydrates: 30g

- Fat: 28g

- Fiber: 8g

Cook Time: None **Prep Time:** 15 minutes *Servings:* 4

Sprouted Quinoa and Avocado Bowl

Ingredients:

- 2 cups cooked sprouted quinoa

- 1 avocado, diced

- 1 cup mixed greens (such as lettuce, spinach, arugula)

- 1/4 cup shredded carrots

- 1/4 cup sliced cucumber

- 1/4 cup chopped red bell pepper

- 2 tablespoons lemon juice

- 2 tablespoons extra-virgin olive oil

- Salt and pepper, to taste

- Optional: pumpkin seeds, sunflower seeds, hemp seeds

Instructions:

1. In a large bowl, combine cooked sprouted quinoa, diced avocado, mixed greens, shredded carrots, sliced cucumber, and chopped red bell pepper.

2. Drizzle with lemon juice and olive oil.

3. Season with salt and pepper to taste.

4. Toss gently until well combined.

5. Serve chilled or at room temperature.

6. Top with pumpkin seeds, sunflower seeds, or hemp seeds, if desired.

Nutritional Info (per serving):

- Calories: 320

- Protein: 8g

- Carbohydrates: 30g

- Fat: 20g

- Fiber: 8g

Cook Time: Varies (depends on the sprouted quinoa) **Prep Time:** 15 minutes
Servings: 4

DINNER RECIPES

Raw Veggie Lasagna

Ingredients:

- 3 medium zucchinis, thinly sliced lengthwise

- 2 cups cashew ricotta (made by blending cashews, lemon juice, nutritional yeast, and salt)

- 2 cups marinara sauce (made with fresh tomatoes, garlic, basil, and olive oil)

- 1 cup sliced mushrooms

- 1 cup spinach leaves

- 1/2 cup sliced bell peppers

- 1/4 cup chopped fresh basil

Instructions:

1. In a lasagna dish, layer zucchini slices, cashew ricotta, marinara sauce, mushrooms, spinach, and bell peppers.

2. Repeat layers until all ingredients are used, finishing with a layer of marinara sauce on top.

3. Sprinkle with chopped basil.

4. Cover and refrigerate for at least 1 hour before serving.

5. Slice and serve chilled.

Nutritional Info (per serving):

- Calories: 250

- Protein: 8g

- Carbohydrates: 18g

- Fat: 18g

- Fiber: 5g

Cook Time: None **Prep Time:** 30 minutes *Servings:* 6

Sprouted Lentil and Vegetable Stew

Ingredients:

- 2 cups sprouted lentils

- 4 cups vegetable broth

- 1 onion, diced

- 2 carrots, diced

- 2 celery stalks, diced

- 2 garlic cloves, minced

- 1 can (14 oz) diced tomatoes

- 1 teaspoon dried thyme

- 1 teaspoon dried rosemary

- Salt and pepper, to taste

- Fresh parsley, for garnish

Instructions:

1. In a large pot, combine sprouted lentils, vegetable broth, onion, carrots, celery, garlic, diced tomatoes, thyme, rosemary, salt, and pepper.

2. Bring to a boil, then reduce heat and simmer for 20-25 minutes, or until lentils and vegetables are tender.

3. Serve hot, garnished with fresh parsley.

Nutritional Info (per serving):

- Calories: 280

- Protein: 18g

- Carbohydrates: 50g

- Fat: 2g

- Fiber: 20g

Cook Time: 25 minutes **Prep Time:** 15 minutes *Servings:* 6

Fermented Cabbage Rolls

Ingredients:

- 12 large cabbage leaves

- 2 cups cooked quinoa

- 1 onion, diced

- 2 garlic cloves, minced

- 1 can (14 oz) diced tomatoes

- 1 teaspoon smoked paprika

- 1 teaspoon dried oregano

- Salt and pepper, to taste

- Fermented sauerkraut

Instructions:

1. Preheat the oven to 350°F (175°C).

2. In a large skillet, sauté onion and garlic until softened.

3. Add cooked quinoa, diced tomatoes, smoked paprika, oregano, salt, and pepper. Cook for another 5 minutes.

4. Place a spoonful of the quinoa mixture onto each cabbage leaf and roll up, tucking in the sides.

5. Place the cabbage rolls in a baking dish, seam side down.

6. Cover with foil and bake for 30 minutes.

7. Serve hot, topped with fermented sauerkraut.

Nutritional Info (per serving):

- Calories: 200

- Protein: 8g

- Carbohydrates: 40g

- Fat: 1g

- Fiber: 10g

Cook Time: 35 minutes **Prep Time:** 30 minutes *Servings:* 6

Raw Zucchini Pasta with Marinara Sauce

Ingredients:

- 3 medium zucchinis, spiralized

- 2 cups cherry tomatoes, halved

- 1/4 cup sun-dried tomatoes, soaked and chopped

- 1/4 cup chopped fresh basil

- 2 tablespoons olive oil

- 1 tablespoon balsamic vinegar

- 1 garlic clove, minced

- Salt and pepper, to taste

Instructions:

1. In a large bowl, combine spiralized zucchini, cherry tomatoes, sun-dried tomatoes, and basil.

2. In a small bowl, whisk together olive oil, balsamic vinegar, garlic, salt, and pepper.

3. Pour the marinara sauce over the zucchini mixture and toss until well coated.

4. Serve immediately.

Nutritional Info (per serving):

- Calories: 150

- Protein: 5g

- Carbohydrates: 20g

- Fat: 7g

- Fiber: 5g

Cook Time: None **Prep Time:** 15 minutes *Servings:* 4

Fresh Herb and Avocado Salad

Ingredients:

- 6 cups mixed salad greens (such as lettuce, spinach, arugula)

- 1/2 cup chopped fresh herbs (such as parsley, cilantro, dill)

- 1 avocado, diced

- 1/4 cup sliced radishes

- 1/4 cup sliced cucumber

- 1/4 cup sliced red onion

- 2 tablespoons lemon juice

- 2 tablespoons olive oil

- Salt and pepper, to taste

Instructions:

1. In a large bowl, combine mixed salad greens, chopped herbs, diced avocado, sliced radishes, sliced cucumber, and sliced red onion.

2. Drizzle with lemon juice and olive oil.

3. Season with salt and pepper to taste.

4. Toss gently until well combined.

5. Serve immediately.

Nutritional Info (per serving):

- Calories: 180

- Protein: 3g

- Carbohydrates: 10g

- Fat: 15g

- Fiber: 5g

Cook Time: None **Prep Time:** 10 minutes *Servings:* 4

Raw Stuffed Bell Peppers

Ingredients:

- 4 large bell peppers, halved and seeds removed

- 2 cups cauliflower florets

- 1/2 cup chopped fresh parsley

- 1/2 cup chopped fresh mint

- 1/4 cup chopped red onion

- 1/4 cup chopped cucumber

- 1/4 cup chopped bell pepper

- 2 tablespoons olive oil

- 2 tablespoons lemon juice

- 1 tablespoon apple cider vinegar

- 1 clove garlic, minced

- Salt and pepper, to taste

Instructions:

1. In a food processor, pulse cauliflower florets until they resemble rice.

2. In a large bowl, combine cauliflower rice, parsley, mint, red onion, cucumber, and bell pepper.

3. In a small bowl, whisk together olive oil, lemon juice, apple cider vinegar, garlic, salt, and pepper.

4. Pour the dressing over the cauliflower mixture and toss until well combined.

5. Serve chilled or at room temperature.

Nutritional Info (per serving):

- Calories: 120

- Protein: 4g

- Carbohydrates: 10g

- Fat: 8g

- Fiber: 4g

Cook Time: None **Prep Time:** 15 minutes *Servings:* 4

Fermented Vegetable Stir-Fry

Ingredients:

- 2 cups mixed fermented vegetables (such as cabbage, carrots, radishes)

- 1 onion, thinly sliced

- 2 garlic cloves, minced

- 1 tablespoon grated ginger

- 2 tablespoons tamari or soy sauce

- 1 tablespoon sesame oil

- 1 tablespoon rice vinegar

- 1 teaspoon maple syrup

- 1 tablespoon olive oil

- Optional: cooked brown rice or quinoa

Instructions:

1. In a large skillet, heat olive oil over medium heat.

2. Add onion, garlic, and ginger. Sauté for 2-3 minutes, until fragrant.

3. Add mixed fermented vegetables and cook for another 3-4 minutes.

4. In a small bowl, whisk together tamari, sesame oil, rice vinegar, and maple syrup.

5. Pour the sauce over the vegetables and stir to combine.

6. Cook for an additional 2-3 minutes.

7. Serve hot over cooked brown rice or quinoa, if desired.

Nutritional Info (per serving, without rice or quinoa):

- Calories: 120

- Protein: 3g

- Carbohydrates: 10g

- Fat: 8g

- Fiber: 4g

Cook Time: 10 minutes **Prep Time:** 10 minutes *Servings:* 4

Raw Kale and Avocado Salad

Ingredients:

- 6 cups chopped kale leaves

- 1 avocado, diced

- 1/4 cup chopped red onion

- 1/4 cup dried cranberries

- 1/4 cup sliced almonds

- 2 tablespoons lemon juice

- 2 tablespoons olive oil

- 1 tablespoon maple syrup

- Salt and pepper, to taste

Instructions:

1. In a large bowl, combine chopped kale, diced avocado, chopped red onion, dried cranberries, and sliced almonds.

2. In a small bowl, whisk together lemon juice, olive oil, maple syrup, salt, and pepper.

3. Pour the dressing over the salad and toss until well coated.

4. Serve immediately.

Nutritional Info (per serving):

- Calories: 250

- Protein: 5g

- Carbohydrates: 22g

- Fat: 18g

- Fiber: 7g

Cook Time: None ***Prep Time:*** 15 minutes *Servings:* 4

Raw Carrot and Ginger Soup

Ingredients:

- 6 large carrots, peeled and chopped

- 1-inch piece of ginger, peeled and chopped

- 1/2 cup raw cashews, soaked for 2 hours and drained

- 4 cups water or vegetable broth

- 2 tablespoons lemon juice

- 1 tablespoon olive oil

- Salt and pepper, to taste

- Optional: fresh cilantro, for garnish

Instructions:

1. In a blender, combine chopped carrots, chopped ginger, soaked cashews, water or vegetable broth, lemon juice, olive oil, salt, and pepper.

2. Blend until smooth and creamy.

3. If the soup is too thick, add more water or broth until desired consistency is reached.

4. Pour the soup into bowls and garnish with fresh cilantro, if desired.

5. Serve chilled or at room temperature.

Nutritional Info (per serving):

- Calories: 180

- Protein: 4g

- Carbohydrates: 20g

- Fat: 10g

- Fiber: 6g

Cook Time: None **Prep Time:** 15 minutes (plus soaking time for cashews) *Servings:* 4

Sprouted Grain and Veggie Burger

Ingredients:

- 1 cup cooked sprouted grains (such as quinoa, millet, or brown rice)

- 1 can (15 oz) black beans, drained and rinsed

- 1/2 cup diced bell peppers

- 1/2 cup diced red onion

- 1/4 cup chopped fresh cilantro

- 1 teaspoon ground cumin

- 1 teaspoon smoked paprika

- Salt and pepper, to taste

- Optional: whole grain burger buns, lettuce, tomato slices, avocado slices

Instructions:

1. In a large bowl, mash black beans with a fork until mostly smooth.

2. Add cooked sprouted grains, diced bell peppers, diced red onion, chopped cilantro, ground cumin, smoked paprika, salt, and pepper. Mix until well combined.

3. Divide the mixture into 4 equal portions and shape into burger patties.

4. Heat a skillet over medium heat and lightly grease with oil.

5. Cook the burger patties for 4-5 minutes per side, or until golden brown and heated through.

6. Serve the burgers on whole grain buns with lettuce, tomato slices, and avocado slices, if desired.

Nutritional Info (per serving, without bun and toppings):

- Calories: 200

- Protein: 9g

- Carbohydrates: 35g

- Fat: 2g

- Fiber: 10g

Cook Time: 10 minutes **Prep Time:** 15 minutes *Servings:* 4

Raw Eggplant and Tomato Stack

Ingredients:

- 1 large eggplant, sliced into rounds

- 2 large tomatoes, sliced into rounds

- 1/2 cup cashew cheese (made by blending cashews, lemon juice, nutritional yeast, and salt)

- 1/4 cup chopped fresh basil

- 1/4 cup balsamic vinegar

- 2 tablespoons olive oil

- Salt and pepper, to taste

Instructions:

1. Preheat the oven to 400°F (200°C).

2. Place eggplant slices on a baking sheet lined with parchment paper.

3. Drizzle with olive oil and season with salt and pepper.

4. Roast in the oven for 20-25 minutes, or until eggplant is tender.

5. In a small bowl, whisk together balsamic vinegar and olive oil to make a dressing.

6. To assemble the stacks, place a slice of eggplant on a plate, followed by a slice of tomato and a spoonful of cashew cheese.

7. Repeat layers until all ingredients are used, finishing with a drizzle of the balsamic dressing.

8. Garnish with chopped basil.

9. Serve immediately.

Nutritional Info (per serving):

- Calories: 180

- Protein: 5g

- Carbohydrates: 15g

- Fat: 12g

- Fiber: 5g

Cook Time: 25 minutes **Prep Time:** 15 minutes *Servings:* 4

Fermented Radish and Cucumber Salad

Ingredients:

- 1 bunch radishes, thinly sliced
- 1 cucumber, thinly sliced
- 2 tablespoons apple cider vinegar
- 1 tablespoon maple syrup
- 1 teaspoon sea salt
- 1/2 teaspoon mustard seeds
- 1/2 teaspoon dill seeds
- 1/4 teaspoon black peppercorns
- 1/4 cup water (if needed)

Instructions:

1. In a large bowl, combine sliced radishes and sliced cucumber.

2. In a small bowl, whisk together apple cider vinegar, maple syrup, sea salt, mustard seeds, dill seeds, and black peppercorns.

3. Pour the dressing over the radish and cucumber mixture and toss until well coated.

4. If the mixture seems dry, add water, 1 tablespoon at a time, until the vegetables are submerged.

5. Transfer the mixture to a clean glass jar, pressing it down firmly to remove any air bubbles and ensure it is submerged in liquid.

6. Cover the jar loosely with a lid or a clean cloth secured with a rubber band.

7. Allow the salad to ferment at room temperature for 3 to 7 days, depending on desired level of fermentation.

8. Once fermented to your liking, transfer the jar to the refrigerator to slow down the fermentation process.

9. Serve chilled as a side dish or topping for salads and sandwiches.

Nutritional Info (per serving):

- Calories: 30

- Protein: 1g

- Carbohydrates: 6g

- Fat: 0g

- Fiber: 2g

Cook Time: None **Prep Time:** 15 minutes *Servings:* 4

Raw Nori Rolls with Vegetables

Ingredients:

- 4 sheets nori seaweed

- 2 cups cooked quinoa

- 1 avocado, thinly sliced

- 1/2 cucumber, julienned

- 1/2 bell pepper, julienned

- 1/4 cup shredded carrots

- 1/4 cup alfalfa sprouts

- Tamari or soy sauce, for dipping

Instructions:

1. Place a nori sheet on a clean, flat surface.

2. Spread a thin layer of quinoa over the nori sheet, leaving about 1 inch of space at the top.

3. Layer avocado slices, cucumber, bell pepper, shredded carrots, and alfalfa sprouts on top of the quinoa.

4. Starting from the bottom, roll the nori sheet tightly, using a little water to seal the edge.

5. Repeat with remaining nori sheets and filling.

6. Slice each roll into bite-sized pieces.

7. Serve with tamari or soy sauce for dipping.

Nutritional Info (per serving):

- Calories: 200

- Protein: 6g

- Carbohydrates: 30g

- Fat: 7g

- Fiber: 7g

Cook Time: None **Prep Time:** 20 minutes *Servings:* 4

Sprouted Bean and Veggie Chili

Ingredients:

- 2 cups cooked sprouted beans (such as kidney beans, black beans, or chickpeas)

- 1 onion, diced

- 2 garlic cloves, minced

- 1 bell pepper, diced

- 1 zucchini, diced

- 1 carrot, diced

- 1 can (14 oz) diced tomatoes

- 2 cups vegetable broth

- 2 tablespoons chili powder

- 1 teaspoon cumin

- Salt and pepper, to taste

- Optional toppings: avocado slices, chopped cilantro, lime wedges

Instructions:

1. In a large pot, sauté onion and garlic until softened.

2. Add diced bell pepper, zucchini, and carrot. Cook for another 5 minutes.

3. Stir in cooked sprouted beans, diced tomatoes, vegetable broth, chili powder, cumin, salt, and pepper.

4. Bring to a boil, then reduce heat and simmer for 20-30 minutes, or until vegetables are tender and flavors have melded.

5. Serve hot, garnished with avocado slices, chopped cilantro, and lime wedges, if desired.

Nutritional Info (per serving):

- Calories: 250

- Protein: 12g

- Carbohydrates: 45g

- Fat: 2g

- Fiber: 15g

Cook Time: 30 minutes **Prep Time:** 15 minutes *Servings:* 4

Raw Sweet Potato and Pecan Salad

Ingredients:

- 2 sweet potatoes, peeled and grated

- 1/2 cup chopped pecans

- 1/4 cup dried cranberries

- 1/4 cup chopped fresh parsley

- 2 tablespoons lemon juice

- 2 tablespoons olive oil

- 1 tablespoon maple syrup

- Salt and pepper, to taste

Instructions:

1. In a large bowl, combine grated sweet potatoes, chopped pecans, dried cranberries, and chopped parsley.

2. In a small bowl, whisk together lemon juice, olive oil, maple syrup, salt, and pepper.

3. Pour the dressing over the sweet potato mixture and toss until well coated.

4. Serve chilled or at room temperature.

Nutritional Info (per serving):

- Calories: 220

- Protein: 3g

- Carbohydrates: 30g

- Fat: 10g

- Fiber: 5g

Cook Time: None **Prep Time:** 15 minutes *Servings:* 4

Fermented Carrot and Beet Salad

Ingredients:

- 2 cups grated carrots

- 2 cups grated beets

- 1 tablespoon sea salt

- 1 teaspoon caraway seeds

- 1/2 teaspoon mustard seeds

- 1/4 teaspoon black peppercorns

- 1/4 cup water (if needed)

Instructions:

1. In a large bowl, combine grated carrots and grated beets.

2. In a small bowl, mix together sea salt, caraway seeds, mustard seeds, and black peppercorns.

3. Sprinkle the salt mixture over the carrots and beets.

4. Massage the vegetables with clean hands for about 5 minutes, or until they start to release their juices.

5. If the mixture seems dry, add water, 1 tablespoon at a time, until the vegetables are submerged.

6. Transfer the mixture to a clean glass jar, pressing it down firmly to remove any air bubbles and ensure it is submerged in liquid.

7. Cover the jar loosely with a lid or a clean cloth secured with a rubber band.

8. Allow the salad to ferment at room temperature for 3 to 7 days, depending on desired level of fermentation.

9. Once fermented to your liking, transfer the jar to the refrigerator to slow down the fermentation process.

10. Serve chilled as a side dish or topping for salads and sandwiches.

Nutritional Info (per serving):

- Calories: 40

- Protein: 1g

- Carbohydrates: 10g

- Fat: 0g

- Fiber: 3g

Cook Time: None **Prep Time:** 15 minutes *Servings:* 4

Raw Broccoli and Almond Stir-Fry

Ingredients:

- 2 cups broccoli florets

- 1/4 cup sliced almonds

- 1/4 cup diced red bell pepper

- 2 tablespoons tamari or soy sauce

- 1 tablespoon sesame oil

- 1 tablespoon rice vinegar

- 1 teaspoon maple syrup

- 1 clove garlic, minced

- 1 teaspoon grated ginger

- Optional: cooked brown rice or quinoa

Instructions:

1. In a large skillet, heat sesame oil over medium heat.

2. Add minced garlic and grated ginger. Sauté for 1-2 minutes, until fragrant.

3. Add broccoli florets, sliced almonds, and diced red bell pepper. Cook for 5-7 minutes, or until vegetables are tender-crisp.

4. In a small bowl, whisk together tamari or soy sauce, rice vinegar, and maple syrup.

5. Pour the sauce over the vegetables and stir to combine.

6. Cook for an additional 2-3 minutes.

7. Serve hot over cooked brown rice or quinoa, if desired.

Nutritional Info (per serving, without rice or quinoa):

- Calories: 120

- Protein: 5g

- Carbohydrates: 10g

- Fat: 8g

- Fiber: 4g

Cook Time: 15 minutes **Prep Time:** 10 minutes *Servings:* 4

Raw Asparagus and Spinach Salad

Ingredients:

- 1 bunch asparagus, trimmed and thinly sliced

- 4 cups baby spinach leaves

- 1/4 cup sliced almonds

- 1/4 cup dried cranberries

- 2 tablespoons lemon juice

- 2 tablespoons olive oil

- 1 tablespoon maple syrup

- Salt and pepper, to taste

Instructions:

1. In a large bowl, combine sliced asparagus, baby spinach leaves, sliced almonds, and dried cranberries.

2. In a small bowl, whisk together lemon juice, olive oil, maple syrup, salt, and pepper.

3. Pour the dressing over the salad and toss until well coated.

4. Serve immediately.

Nutritional Info (per serving):

- Calories: 180

- Protein: 5g

- Carbohydrates: 20g

- Fat: 10g

- Fiber: 6g

Cook Time: None **Prep Time:** 15 minutes *Servings:* 4

Sprouted Lentil and Veggie Bowl

Ingredients:

- 2 cups cooked sprouted lentils

- 1 bell pepper, diced

- 1 cucumber, diced

- 1 carrot, shredded

- 1/4 cup chopped fresh parsley

- 2 tablespoons lemon juice

- 2 tablespoons olive oil

- Salt and pepper, to taste

- Optional: avocado slices, sesame seeds

Instructions:

1. In a large bowl, combine cooked sprouted lentils, diced bell pepper, diced cucumber, shredded carrot, and chopped parsley.

2. In a small bowl, whisk together lemon juice, olive oil, salt, and pepper.

3. Pour the dressing over the lentil and veggie mixture and toss until well combined.

4. Serve chilled or at room temperature.

5. Garnish with avocado slices and sesame seeds, if desired.

Nutritional Info (per serving):

- Calories: 250
- Protein: 12g
- Carbohydrates: 30g
- Fat: 10g
- Fiber: 10g

Cook Time: None **Prep Time:** 15 minutes *Servings:* 4

Raw Cabbage and Apple Slaw

Ingredients:

- 1/2 head green cabbage, thinly sliced
- 1 apple, julienned
- 1/4 cup chopped fresh cilantro
- 1/4 cup chopped fresh mint
- 2 tablespoons apple cider vinegar
- 1 tablespoon olive oil
- 1 teaspoon maple syrup
- Salt and pepper, to taste

Instructions:

1. In a large bowl, combine thinly sliced green cabbage, julienned apple, chopped cilantro, and chopped mint.

2. In a small bowl, whisk together apple cider vinegar, olive oil, maple syrup, salt, and pepper.

3. Pour the dressing over the cabbage and apple mixture and toss until well coated.

4. Serve chilled or at room temperature.

Nutritional Info (per serving):

- Calories: 100
- Protein: 2g
- Carbohydrates: 15g
- Fat: 5g

- Fiber: 5g

Cook Time: None **Prep Time:** 15 minutes *Servings:* 4

Fermented Kimchi and Tofu Stir-Fry

Ingredients:

- 2 cups fermented kimchi

- 1 block (14 oz) firm tofu, diced

- 1 onion, sliced

- 2 garlic cloves, minced

- 1 tablespoon grated ginger

- 2 tablespoons soy sauce

- 1 tablespoon sesame oil

- 1 tablespoon rice vinegar

- 1 teaspoon maple syrup

- 2 green onions, sliced

- Optional: cooked brown rice

Instructions:

1. In a large skillet, heat sesame oil over medium heat.

2. Add sliced onion, minced garlic, and grated ginger. Sauté for 2-3 minutes, until fragrant.

3. Add diced tofu and soy sauce. Cook for another 5 minutes, stirring occasionally.

4. Add fermented kimchi, rice vinegar, and maple syrup. Cook for an additional 5 minutes.

5. Serve hot, garnished with sliced green onions.

6. Serve over cooked brown rice, if desired.

Nutritional Info (per serving, without rice):

- Calories: 200

- Protein: 15g

- Carbohydrates: 15g

- Fat: 10g

- Fiber: 5g

Cook Time: 15 minutes **Prep Time:** 10 minutes *Servings:* 4

Raw Mushroom and Walnut Tacos

Ingredients:

- 8 large mushroom caps

- 1/2 cup walnuts

- 1/4 cup chopped fresh cilantro

- 1/4 cup chopped red onion

- 1/4 cup diced bell pepper

- 2 tablespoons lime juice

- 1 tablespoon olive oil

- 1 teaspoon chili powder

- 1/2 teaspoon cumin

- Salt and pepper, to taste

- 4 large lettuce leaves

Instructions:

1. In a food processor, pulse mushroom caps and walnuts until finely chopped.

2. Transfer the mixture to a large bowl and add chopped cilantro, red onion, bell pepper, lime juice, olive oil, chili powder, cumin, salt, and pepper. Mix until well combined.

3. Spoon the mixture onto lettuce leaves, dividing evenly.

4. Serve immediately.

Nutritional Info (per serving):

- Calories: 150

- Protein: 5g

- Carbohydrates: 8g

- Fat: 12g

- Fiber: 3g

Cook Time: None *Prep Time:* 15 minutes *Servings:* 4

Sprouted Grain and Veggie Wraps

Ingredients:

- 4 large sprouted grain wraps
- 1 avocado, mashed
- 1 cup mixed greens
- 1/2 cup shredded carrots
- 1/2 cup sliced cucumber
- 1/2 cup sliced bell pepper
- 1/4 cup hummus
- 2 tablespoons lemon juice
- Salt and pepper, to taste

Instructions:

1. Lay out the sprouted grain wraps on a clean surface.
2. Spread mashed avocado evenly over each wrap.
3. Top with mixed greens, shredded carrots, sliced cucumber, and sliced bell pepper.
4. Drizzle with hummus and lemon juice.
5. Season with salt and pepper.
6. Roll up the wraps tightly and slice in half.
7. Serve immediately.

Nutritional Info (per serving):

- Calories: 250

- Protein: 8g

- Carbohydrates: 30g

- Fat: 12g

- Fiber: 10g

Cook Time: None **Prep Time:** 15 minutes *Servings:* 4

Raw Red Pepper and Avocado Salad

Ingredients:

- 2 red bell peppers, thinly sliced

- 1 avocado, diced

- 1/4 cup chopped fresh cilantro

- 2 tablespoons lime juice

- 1 tablespoon olive oil

- Salt and pepper, to taste

Instructions:

1. In a large bowl, combine thinly sliced red bell peppers, diced avocado, chopped cilantro, lime juice, olive oil, salt, and pepper.

2. Toss until well coated.

3. Serve chilled or at room temperature.

Nutritional Info (per serving):

- Calories: 150

- Protein: 2g

- Carbohydrates: 12g

- Fat: 12g

- Fiber: 6g

Cook Time: None **Prep Time:** 10 minutes *Servings:* 4

Fermented Carrot and Ginger Soup

Ingredients:

- 6 large carrots, peeled and chopped

- 1-inch piece of ginger, peeled and chopped

- 1/2 cup raw cashews, soaked for 2 hours and drained

- 4 cups water or vegetable broth

- 2 tablespoons lemon juice

- 1 tablespoon olive oil

- Salt and pepper, to taste

- Optional: fresh cilantro, for garnish

Instructions:

1. In a blender, combine chopped carrots, chopped ginger, soaked cashews, water or vegetable broth, lemon juice, olive oil, salt, and pepper.

2. Blend until smooth and creamy.

3. If the soup is too thick, add more water or broth until desired consistency is reached.

4. Pour the soup into bowls and garnish with fresh cilantro, if desired.

5. Serve chilled or at room temperature.

Nutritional Info (per serving):

- Calories: 180

- Protein: 4g

- Carbohydrates: 20g

- Fat: 10g

- Fiber: 6g

Cook Time: None **Prep Time:** 15 minutes (plus soaking time for cashews) *Servings:* 4

Raw Cauliflower and Broccoli Salad

Ingredients:

- 1 head cauliflower, chopped into florets

- 1 head broccoli, chopped into florets

- 1/4 cup chopped red onion

- 1/4 cup chopped fresh parsley

- 2 tablespoons lemon juice

- 2 tablespoons olive oil

- Salt and pepper, to taste

Instructions:

1. In a large bowl, combine chopped cauliflower, chopped broccoli, chopped red onion, and chopped parsley.

2. In a small bowl, whisk together lemon juice, olive oil, salt, and pepper.

3. Pour the dressing over the cauliflower and broccoli mixture and toss until well coated.

4. Serve chilled or at room temperature.

Nutritional Info (per serving):

- Calories: 150
- Protein: 6g
- Carbohydrates: 20g
- Fat: 7g
- Fiber: 10g

Cook Time: None **Prep Time:** 15 minutes *Servings:* 4

Sprouted Quinoa and Veggie Bowl

Ingredients:

- 2 cups cooked sprouted quinoa
- 1 bell pepper, diced
- 1 cucumber, diced
- 1 carrot, shredded
- 1/4 cup chopped fresh cilantro
- 2 tablespoons lime juice
- 2 tablespoons olive oil
- Salt and pepper, to taste
- Optional: avocado slices, sesame seeds

Instructions:

1. In a large bowl, combine cooked sprouted quinoa, diced bell pepper, diced cucumber, shredded carrot, chopped cilantro, lime juice, olive oil, salt, and pepper.

2. Toss until well combined.

3. Serve chilled or at room temperature.

4. Garnish with avocado slices and sesame seeds, if desired.

Nutritional Info (per serving):

- Calories: 250

- Protein: 10g

- Carbohydrates: 30g

- Fat: 10g

- Fiber: 8g

Cook Time: None **Prep Time:** 15 minutes *Servings:* 4

Raw Carrot and Cashew Curry

Ingredients:

- 4 large carrots, peeled and chopped

- 1/2 cup raw cashews, soaked for 2 hours and drained

- 1 can (14 oz) coconut milk

- 2 tablespoons curry powder

- 1 tablespoon grated ginger

- 1 tablespoon coconut oil

- Salt and pepper, to taste

- Optional: cooked brown rice

Instructions:

1. In a blender, combine chopped carrots, soaked cashews, coconut milk, curry powder, and grated ginger.

2. Blend until smooth.

3. In a large skillet, heat coconut oil over medium heat.

4. Pour the carrot-cashew mixture into the skillet and cook for 10-15 minutes, stirring occasionally, until heated through and slightly thickened.

5. Season with salt and pepper.

6. Serve hot over cooked brown rice, if desired.

Nutritional Info (per serving, without rice):

- Calories: 250

- Protein: 6g

- Carbohydrates: 20g

- Fat: 18g

- Fiber: 6g

Cook Time: 15 minutes **Prep Time:** 15 minutes (plus soaking time for cashews) *Servings:* 4

SNACKS RECIPES

Raw Energy Balls with Dates and Nuts

Ingredients:

- 1 cup pitted dates

- 1 cup mixed nuts (such as almonds, cashews, and walnuts)

- 2 tablespoons raw cacao powder

- 1/2 teaspoon vanilla extract

- Pinch of salt

- Optional: shredded coconut, cocoa powder, or chopped nuts for coating

Instructions:

1. In a food processor, blend dates, mixed nuts, cacao powder, vanilla extract, and salt until a sticky dough forms.

2. Roll the dough into small balls.

3. If desired, roll the balls in shredded coconut, cocoa powder, or chopped nuts for coating.

4. Refrigerate for at least 30 minutes before serving.

Nutritional Info (per serving):

- Calories: 100

- Protein: 2g

- Carbohydrates: 12g

- Fat: 6g

- Fiber: 2g

Cook Time: None **Prep Time:** 15 minutes *Servings:* 12 balls

Sprouted Seed Crackers

Ingredients:

- 1 cup sprouted seeds (such as sunflower seeds, pumpkin seeds, and sesame seeds)

- 1/4 cup ground flaxseeds

- 1/4 cup water

- 1/2 teaspoon salt

- 1/2 teaspoon garlic powder

- 1/2 teaspoon onion powder

- 1/2 teaspoon dried herbs (such as thyme or rosemary)

Instructions:

1. Preheat the oven to 325°F (165°C) and line a baking sheet with parchment paper.

2. In a bowl, combine sprouted seeds, ground flaxseeds, water, salt, garlic powder, onion powder, and dried herbs. Mix well.

3. Spread the mixture onto the prepared baking sheet, pressing it into a thin, even layer.

4. Bake for 25-30 minutes, or until crisp and golden.

5. Remove from the oven and let cool completely before breaking into pieces.

Nutritional Info (per serving):

- Calories: 100

- Protein: 4g

- Carbohydrates: 4g

- Fat: 8g

- Fiber: 3g

Cook Time: 30 minutes **Prep Time:** 10 minutes *Servings:* 4

Fermented Vegetable Chips

Ingredients:

- Assorted vegetables (such as carrots, beets, sweet potatoes, and parsnips), thinly sliced

- Fermented vegetable brine or whey

- Salt

Instructions:

1. Preheat the oven to 200°F (95°C) and line a baking sheet with parchment paper.

2. Dip the vegetable slices in fermented vegetable brine or whey, then arrange them on the prepared baking sheet.

3. Sprinkle with salt.

4. Bake for 2-3 hours, or until crispy, flipping halfway through.

5. Let cool before serving.

Nutritional Info (per serving):

- Calories: 50

- Protein: 1g

- Carbohydrates: 10g

- Fat: 1g

- Fiber: 2g

Cook Time: 2-3 hours *Prep Time:* 15 minutes *Servings:* 4

Raw Almond Butter and Apple Slices

Ingredients:

- 2 apples, cored and sliced

- 1/4 cup raw almond butter

Instructions:

1. Spread almond butter on apple slices.

2. Serve immediately.

Nutritional Info (per serving):

- Calories: 200

- Protein: 4g

- Carbohydrates: 20g

- Fat: 12g

- Fiber: 5g

Cook Time: None *Prep Time:* 5 minutes *Servings:* 2

Sprouted Hummus with Veggie Sticks

Ingredients:

- 1 cup sprouted chickpeas
- 2 tablespoons tahini
- 2 tablespoons lemon juice
- 1 garlic clove, minced
- 1/2 teaspoon ground cumin
- Salt and pepper, to taste
- Assorted vegetable sticks (such as carrots, cucumbers, and bell peppers), for serving

Instructions:

1. In a food processor, combine sprouted chickpeas, tahini, lemon juice, garlic clove, cumin, salt, and pepper. Blend until smooth.
2. Serve the hummus with assorted vegetable sticks.

Nutritional Info (per serving):

- Calories: 150
- Protein: 5g
- Carbohydrates: 15g
- Fat: 8g
- Fiber: 5g

Cook Time: None **Prep Time:** 10 minutes *Servings:* 4

Raw Coconut Macaroons

Ingredients:

- 2 cups shredded coconut

- 1/2 cup coconut oil, melted

- 1/4 cup maple syrup

- 1 teaspoon vanilla extract

- Pinch of salt

Instructions:

1. Preheat the oven to 325°F (165°C) and line a baking sheet with parchment paper.

2. In a large bowl, combine shredded coconut, melted coconut oil, maple syrup, vanilla extract, and salt. Mix well.

3. Using a cookie scoop or spoon, drop rounded tablespoons of the mixture onto the prepared baking sheet.

4. Bake for 15-20 minutes, or until golden brown.

5. Remove from the oven and let cool completely before serving.

Nutritional Info (per serving):

- Calories: 200

- Protein: 1g

- Carbohydrates: 10g

- Fat: 18g

- Fiber: 3g

Cook Time: 15-20 minutes **Prep Time:** 10 minutes *Servings:* 12 macaroons

Fermented Cabbage and Carrot Rolls

Ingredients:

- 1 head cabbage, leaves separated
- 2 carrots, grated
- Fermented vegetable brine or whey

Instructions:

1. Place a cabbage leaf on a clean surface.
2. Spoon some grated carrots onto the cabbage leaf.
3. Roll up the cabbage leaf, tucking in the sides as you go.
4. Place the roll in a clean glass jar.
5. Repeat with the remaining cabbage leaves and grated carrots.
6. Pour enough fermented vegetable brine or whey over the rolls to cover them completely.
7. Cover the jar loosely with a lid or a clean cloth secured with a rubber band.
8. Allow the rolls to ferment at room temperature for 3-7 days, depending on desired level of fermentation.
9. Once fermented to your liking, transfer the jar to the refrigerator to slow down the fermentation process.
10. Serve chilled as a side dish or snack.

Nutritional Info (per serving):

- Calories: 30
- Protein: 1g

- Carbohydrates: 7g

- Fat: 0g

- Fiber: 3g

Cook Time: None **Prep Time:** 30 minutes *Servings:* 6 rolls

---

Raw Cashew and Raisin Clusters

Ingredients:

- 1 cup raw cashews

- 1/2 cup raisins

Instructions:

1. In a bowl, combine raw cashews and raisins.

2. Mix well.

3. Using your hands, form the mixture into clusters.

4. Refrigerate for at least 30 minutes before serving.

Nutritional Info (per serving):

- Calories: 150

- Protein: 5g

- Carbohydrates: 15g

- Fat: 8g

- Fiber: 2g

Cook Time: None **Prep Time:** 5 minutes *Servings:* 4

Sprouted Lentil Hummus

Ingredients:

- 1 cup sprouted lentils
- 2 tablespoons tahini
- 2 tablespoons lemon juice
- 1 garlic clove, minced
- 1/2 teaspoon ground cumin
- Salt and pepper, to taste
- Water, as needed

Instructions:

1. In a food processor, combine sprouted lentils, tahini, lemon juice, garlic clove, cumin, salt, and pepper. Blend until smooth.
2. If the mixture is too thick, add water, 1 tablespoon at a time, until desired consistency is reached.
3. Serve with veggie sticks or as a spread.

Nutritional Info (per serving):

- Calories: 150
- Protein: 5g
- Carbohydrates: 15g
- Fat: 8g
- Fiber: 5g

Cook Time: None **Prep Time:** 10 minutes *Servings:* 4

Raw Kale Chips

Ingredients:

- 1 bunch kale, stems removed and leaves torn into bite-sized pieces

- 2 tablespoons olive oil

- 1 tablespoon nutritional yeast

- 1 teaspoon garlic powder

- 1/2 teaspoon salt

Instructions:

1. Preheat the oven to 300°F (150°C) and line a baking sheet with parchment paper.

2. In a large bowl, combine kale leaves, olive oil, nutritional yeast, garlic powder, and salt. Massage the kale leaves until well coated.

3. Spread the kale leaves in a single layer on the prepared baking sheet.

4. Bake for 10-15 minutes, or until crisp.

5. Remove from the oven and let cool before serving.

Nutritional Info (per serving):

- Calories: 100

- Protein: 5g

- Carbohydrates: 10g

- Fat: 5g

- Fiber: 5g

Cook Time: 10-15 minutes **Prep Time:** 10 minutes *Servings:* 4

Raw Carrot and Ginger Bites

Ingredients:

- 2 carrots, peeled and chopped
- 1/2 cup almonds
- 1/4 cup shredded coconut
- 1 tablespoon grated ginger
- 1 tablespoon honey or maple syrup
- Pinch of salt

Instructions:

1. In a food processor, combine carrots, almonds, shredded coconut, grated ginger, honey or maple syrup, and salt. Process until well combined and sticky.
2. Roll the mixture into small balls.
3. Refrigerate for at least 30 minutes before serving.

Nutritional Info (per serving):

- Calories: 100
- Protein: 3g
- Carbohydrates: 10g
- Fat: 6g
- Fiber: 3g

Cook Time: None **Prep Time:** 15 minutes *Servings:* 4

Sprouted Nut and Seed Mix

Ingredients:

- 1 cup mixed sprouted nuts and seeds (such as almonds, cashews, sunflower seeds, and pumpkin seeds)
- 1/2 teaspoon salt
- 1/2 teaspoon garlic powder
- 1/2 teaspoon onion powder
- 1/2 teaspoon smoked paprika

Instructions:

1. In a bowl, combine mixed sprouted nuts and seeds, salt, garlic powder, onion powder, and smoked paprika. Mix well.
2. Serve as a snack or topping for salads and soups.

Nutritional Info (per serving):

- Calories: 200
- Protein: 8g
- Carbohydrates: 10g
- Fat: 15g
- Fiber: 5g

Cook Time: None **Prep Time:** 5 minutes *Servings:* 4

Raw Zucchini Chips

Ingredients:

- 2 zucchinis, thinly sliced
- 2 tablespoons olive oil
- 1 tablespoon nutritional yeast
- 1 teaspoon garlic powder
- 1/2 teaspoon salt

Instructions:

1. Preheat the oven to 200°F (95°C) and line a baking sheet with parchment paper.
2. In a large bowl, combine zucchini slices, olive oil, nutritional yeast, garlic powder, and salt. Toss until well coated.
3. Spread the zucchini slices in a single layer on the prepared baking sheet.
4. Bake for 2-3 hours, or until crispy, flipping halfway through.
5. Remove from the oven and let cool before serving.

Nutritional Info (per serving):

- Calories: 100
- Protein: 3g
- Carbohydrates: 5g
- Fat: 8g
- Fiber: 2g

Cook Time: 2-3 hours **Prep Time:** 10 minutes *Servings:* 4

Fermented Radish Slices

Ingredients:

- 1 bunch radishes, thinly sliced
- Fermented vegetable brine or whey
- Salt

Instructions:

1. Place radish slices in a clean glass jar.
2. Pour enough fermented vegetable brine or whey over the radish slices to cover them completely.
3. Add a pinch of salt.
4. Cover the jar loosely with a lid or a clean cloth secured with a rubber band.
5. Allow the radishes to ferment at room temperature for 3-7 days, depending on desired level of fermentation.
6. Once fermented to your liking, transfer the jar to the refrigerator to slow down the fermentation process.
7. Serve chilled as a side dish or snack.

Nutritional Info (per serving):

- Calories: 30
- Protein: 1g
- Carbohydrates: 7g
- Fat: 0g
- Fiber: 2g

Cook Time: None **Prep Time:** 15 minutes *Servings:* 4

Raw Cucumber and Avocado Rolls

Ingredients:

- 1 cucumber

- 1 avocado

- 1/2 red bell pepper, julienned

- 1/4 cup shredded carrots

- 1/4 cup alfalfa sprouts

- 1 tablespoon sesame seeds

- 1 tablespoon soy sauce or tamari

- 1 teaspoon rice vinegar

- 1 teaspoon sesame oil

- Pinch of salt and pepper

Instructions:

1. Using a vegetable peeler or a mandoline, slice the cucumber lengthwise into thin strips.

2. Peel and pit the avocado, then slice it into thin strips.

3. Lay a cucumber strip flat on a clean surface and place a few avocado slices, red bell pepper strips, shredded carrots, and alfalfa sprouts at one end.

4. Roll up the cucumber strip tightly around the filling to form a roll.

5. Repeat with the remaining cucumber strips and filling ingredients.

6. In a small bowl, whisk together sesame seeds, soy sauce or tamari, rice vinegar, sesame oil, salt, and pepper.

7. Drizzle the sauce over the cucumber rolls before serving.

Nutritional Info (per serving):

- Calories: 150

- Protein: 3g

- Carbohydrates: 10g

- Fat: 12g

- Fiber: 5g

Cook Time: None **Prep Time:** 15 minutes *Servings:* 4

Sprouted Chickpea Snacks

Ingredients:

- 1 cup sprouted chickpeas

- 1 tablespoon olive oil

- 1 teaspoon smoked paprika

- 1/2 teaspoon garlic powder

- 1/2 teaspoon salt

Instructions:

1. Preheat the oven to 400°F (200°C) and line a baking sheet with parchment paper.

2. In a bowl, toss sprouted chickpeas with olive oil, smoked paprika, garlic powder, and salt until well coated.

3. Spread the chickpeas in a single layer on the prepared baking sheet.

4. Bake for 20-25 minutes, or until crispy, shaking the pan halfway through.

5. Remove from the oven and let cool before serving.

Nutritional Info (per serving):

- Calories: 100

- Protein: 4g

- Carbohydrates: 12g

- Fat: 4g

- Fiber: 4g

Cook Time: 20-25 minutes **Prep Time:** 5 minutes (plus sprouting time) *Servings:* 4

Raw Coconut and Almond Bars

Ingredients:

- 1 cup almonds

- 1 cup shredded coconut

- 1/2 cup dates, pitted

- 1/4 cup coconut oil, melted

- 1/2 teaspoon vanilla extract

- Pinch of salt

Instructions:

1. In a food processor, blend almonds, shredded coconut, dates, coconut oil, vanilla extract, and salt until a sticky dough forms.

2. Press the dough into a square baking dish lined with parchment paper.

3. Refrigerate for at least 1 hour, or until firm.

4. Cut into bars before serving.

Nutritional Info (per serving):

- Calories: 200

- Protein: 4g

- Carbohydrates: 15g

- Fat: 15g

- Fiber: 5g

Cook Time: None **Prep Time:** 15 minutes (plus chilling time) *Servings:* 8 bars

---

Fermented Beet Chips

Ingredients:

- 2 beets, thinly sliced

- Fermented vegetable brine or whey

- Salt

Instructions:

1. Preheat the oven to 325°F (165°C) and line a baking sheet with parchment paper.

2. Dip the beet slices in fermented vegetable brine or whey, then arrange them on the prepared baking sheet.

3. Sprinkle with salt.

4. Bake for 25-30 minutes, or until crispy, flipping halfway through.

5. Let cool before serving.

Nutritional Info (per serving):

- Calories: 50

- Protein: 1g

- Carbohydrates: 10g

- Fat: 0g

- Fiber: 3g

Cook Time: 25-30 minutes **Prep Time:** 15 minutes *Servings:* 4

Raw Apple and Cinnamon Chips

Ingredients:

- 2 apples, thinly sliced

- 1 tablespoon lemon juice

- 1 teaspoon ground cinnamon

Instructions:

1. Preheat the oven to 200°F (95°C) and line a baking sheet with parchment paper.

2. In a bowl, toss apple slices with lemon juice and ground cinnamon until well coated.

3. Arrange the apple slices in a single layer on the prepared baking sheet.

4. Bake for 1-2 hours, or until dried and crispy, flipping halfway through.

5. Let cool before serving.

Nutritional Info (per serving):

- Calories: 50

- Protein: 0g

- Carbohydrates: 15g

- Fat: 0g

- Fiber: 3g

Cook Time: 1-2 hours **Prep Time:** 10 minutes *Servings:* 4

Sprouted Flax Crackers

Ingredients:

- 1 cup ground flaxseeds

- 1/2 cup water

- 1/2 teaspoon salt

- 1/2 teaspoon garlic powder

- 1/2 teaspoon onion powder

- 1/2 teaspoon dried herbs (such as thyme or rosemary)

Instructions:

1. Preheat the oven to 325°F (165°C) and line a baking sheet with parchment paper.

2. In a bowl, combine ground flaxseeds, water, salt, garlic powder, onion powder, and dried herbs. Mix well.

3. Spread the mixture onto the prepared baking sheet, pressing it into a thin, even layer.

4. Bake for 25-30 minutes, or until firm and crisp.

5. Remove from the oven and let cool before breaking into pieces.

Nutritional Info (per serving):

- Calories: 100

- Protein: 3g

- Carbohydrates: 5g

- Fat: 8g

- Fiber: 4g

Cook Time: 25-30 minutes **Prep Time:** 5 minutes *Servings:* 4

Raw Veggie and Herb Dip

Ingredients:

- 1 cup cashews, soaked for 2 hours and drained

- 1/4 cup water

- 2 tablespoons lemon juice

- 1 garlic clove

- 1/4 cup mixed fresh herbs (such as parsley, dill, and chives)

- Salt and pepper, to taste

Instructions:

1. In a blender, combine soaked cashews, water, lemon juice, garlic clove, mixed fresh herbs, salt, and pepper. Blend until smooth.

2. Serve as a dip for veggie sticks.

Nutritional Info (per serving):

- Calories: 150

- Protein: 5g

- Carbohydrates: 10g

- Fat: 10g

- Fiber: 2g

Cook Time: None **Prep Time:** 10 minutes (plus soaking time for cashews) *Servings:* 4

Fermented Kimchi Bites

Ingredients:

- 1 cup chopped kimchi

- 1/2 cup cooked rice

- 1 tablespoon sesame oil

- 1 teaspoon soy sauce or tamari

- 1 green onion, chopped

- Sesame seeds, for garnish

Instructions:

1. In a bowl, combine chopped kimchi, cooked rice, sesame oil, soy sauce or tamari, and chopped green onion. Mix well.

2. Using your hands, form the mixture into small balls or bites.

3. Place the bites on a plate and sprinkle with sesame seeds.

4. Serve chilled or at room temperature.

Nutritional Info (per serving):

- Calories: 100

- Protein: 2g

- Carbohydrates: 15g

- Fat: 4g

- Fiber: 2g

Cook Time: None **Prep Time:** 10 minutes *Servings:* 4

Raw Banana and Nut Bites

Ingredients:

- 2 bananas, mashed

- 1/2 cup mixed nuts (such as almonds, cashews, and walnuts), chopped

- 1/4 cup shredded coconut

Instructions:

1. In a bowl, combine mashed bananas, chopped mixed nuts, shredded coconut, and cinnamon. Mix well.

2. Using your hands, form the mixture into small bites.

3. Refrigerate for at least 30 minutes before serving.

Nutritional Info (per serving):

- Calories: 150

- Protein: 3g

- Carbohydrates: 20g

- Fat: 8g

- Fiber: 3g

Cook Time: None **Prep Time:** 10 minutes (plus chilling time) *Servings:* 4

Sprouted Pumpkin Seed Mix

Ingredients:

- 1 cup sprouted pumpkin seeds

- 1/2 teaspoon salt

- 1/2 teaspoon garlic powder

- 1/2 teaspoon onion powder

- 1/2 teaspoon smoked paprika

Instructions:

1. In a bowl, combine sprouted pumpkin seeds, salt, garlic powder, onion powder, and smoked paprika. Mix well.

2. Serve as a snack or topping for salads and soups.

Nutritional Info (per serving):

- Calories: 200

- Protein: 10g

- Carbohydrates: 5g

- Fat: 15g

- Fiber: 5g

Cook Time: None **Prep Time:** 5 minutes *Servings:* 4

Raw Veggie Sushi Rolls

Ingredients:

- 2 nori sheets

- 1/2 cucumber, julienned

- 1/2 avocado, sliced

- 1/2 carrot, julienned

- 1/4 red bell pepper, julienned

- 1/4 cup alfalfa sprouts

- Soy sauce or tamari, for dipping

Instructions:

1. Place a nori sheet on a sushi rolling mat or a clean kitchen towel.

2. Arrange cucumber, avocado, carrot, red bell pepper, and alfalfa sprouts in a line along the edge of the nori sheet.

3. Roll up the nori sheet tightly, using the mat or towel to help.

4. Slice the roll into bite-sized pieces.

5. Serve with soy sauce or tamari for dipping.

Nutritional Info (per serving):

- Calories: 100

- Protein: 3g

- Carbohydrates: 10g

- Fat: 6g

- Fiber: 5g

Cook Time: None **Prep Time:** 15 minutes *Servings:* 2 rolls

---

Fermented Pickle Slices

Ingredients:

- 4 cucumbers, thinly sliced

- 2 cups water

- 2 tablespoons salt

- 1 tablespoon dill seeds

- 1 tablespoon mustard seeds

- 1 tablespoon black peppercorns

Instructions:

1. In a large bowl, combine water and salt. Stir until the salt is dissolved.

2. Place cucumber slices, dill seeds, mustard seeds, and black peppercorns in a clean glass jar.

3. Pour the salt water over the cucumber slices, making sure they are completely submerged.

4. Cover the jar loosely with a lid or a clean cloth secured with a rubber band.

5. Allow the pickles to ferment at room temperature for 3-7 days, depending on desired level of fermentation.

6. Once fermented to your liking, transfer the jar to the refrigerator to slow down the fermentation process.

7. Serve chilled as a snack or side dish.

Nutritional Info (per serving):

- Calories: 10

- Protein: 0g

- Carbohydrates: 2g

- Fat: 0g

- Fiber: 1g

Cook Time: None **Prep Time:** 15 minutes *Servings:* 8

Raw Carrot and Nut Pâté

Ingredients:

- 2 carrots, chopped

- 1/2 cup mixed nuts (such as almonds, cashews, and walnuts)

- 1 tablespoon olive oil

- 1 tablespoon lemon juice

- 1 garlic clove

- Pinch of salt and pepper

Instructions:

1. In a food processor, combine chopped carrots, mixed nuts, olive oil, lemon juice, garlic clove, salt, and pepper. Process until smooth.

2. Serve as a spread or dip for veggie sticks.

Nutritional Info (per serving):

- Calories: 100

- Protein: 3g

- Carbohydrates: 7g

- Fat: 8g

- Fiber: 2g

Cook Time: None **Prep Time:** 10 minutes *Servings:* 4

Sprouted Almond and Date Bars

Ingredients:

- 1 cup sprouted almonds

- 1 cup dates, pitted

- 1/4 cup almond butter

- 1/4 cup shredded coconut

- 1/2 teaspoon cinnamon

- Pinch of salt

Instructions:

1. In a food processor, combine sprouted almonds, dates, almond butter, shredded coconut, cinnamon, and salt. Process until a sticky dough forms.

2. Press the dough into a square baking dish lined with parchment paper.

3. Refrigerate for at least 1 hour, or until firm.

4. Cut into bars before serving.

Nutritional Info (per serving):

- Calories: 200

- Protein: 5g

- Carbohydrates: 25g

- Fat: 10g

- Fiber: 5g

Cook Time: None **Prep Time:** 15 minutes (plus chilling time) *Servings:* 8 bars

---

Raw Cabbage and Apple Slaw Bites

Ingredients:

- 1 cup shredded cabbage

- 1 apple, julienned

- 2 tablespoons apple cider vinegar

- 1 tablespoon olive oil

- 1 teaspoon honey

- 1/2 teaspoon caraway seeds

- Pinch of salt and pepper

Instructions:

1. In a bowl, combine shredded cabbage, julienned apple, apple cider vinegar, olive oil, honey, caraway seeds, salt, and pepper. Mix well.

2. Serve as a side dish or snack.

Nutritional Info (per serving):

- Calories: 50

- Protein: 0g

- Carbohydrates: 10g

- Fat: 2g

- Fiber: 2g

Cook Time: None **Prep Time:** 10 minutes *Servings:* 4

Fermented Turnip Chips

Ingredients:

- 2 turnips, thinly sliced

- Fermented vegetable brine or whey

- Salt

Instructions:

1. Preheat the oven to 325°F (165°C) and line a baking sheet with parchment paper.

2. Dip the turnip slices in fermented vegetable brine or whey, then arrange them on the prepared baking sheet.

3. Sprinkle with salt.

4. Bake for 25-30 minutes, or until crispy, flipping halfway through.

5. Let cool before serving.

Nutritional Info (per serving):

- Calories: 50

- Protein: 1g

- Carbohydrates: 10g

- Fat: 0g

- Fiber: 3g

Cook Time: 25-30 minutes ***Prep Time:*** 15 minutes *Servings:* 4

SMOOTHIES RECIPES

Green Detox Smoothie

Ingredients:

- 1 cup spinach

- 1/2 cucumber, peeled and chopped

- 1/2 green apple, cored and chopped

- 1/2 lemon, juiced

- 1 tablespoon fresh ginger, peeled and chopped

- 1 cup coconut water

- Ice cubes (optional)

Instructions:

1. Place spinach, cucumber, apple, lemon juice, ginger, and coconut water in a blender.

2. Blend until smooth.

3. Add ice cubes if desired and blend again until smooth.

4. Pour into a glass and serve.

Nutritional Info (per serving):

- Calories: 70

- Protein: 2g

- Carbohydrates: 16g

- Fat: 1g

- Fiber: 4g

Cook Time: None **Prep Time:** 5 minutes *Servings:* 1

Berry Antioxidant Smoothie

Ingredients:

- 1/2 cup mixed berries (such as strawberries, blueberries, and raspberries)

- 1/2 banana

- 1/2 cup almond milk

- 1 tablespoon chia seeds

- 1 tablespoon honey or maple syrup

Instructions:

1. Place mixed berries, banana, almond milk, chia seeds, and honey or maple syrup in a blender.

2. Blend until smooth.

3. Pour into a glass and serve.

Nutritional Info (per serving):

- Calories: 150

- Protein: 3g

- Carbohydrates: 30g

- Fat: 4g

- Fiber: 8g

Cook Time: None **Prep Time:** 5 minutes *Servings:* 1

Tropical Mango and Pineapple Smoothie

Ingredients:

- 1/2 cup chopped mango
- 1/2 cup chopped pineapple
- 1/2 banana
- 1/2 cup coconut water
- Ice cubes (optional)

Instructions:

1. Place mango, pineapple, banana, and coconut water in a blender.
2. Blend until smooth.
3. Add ice cubes if desired and blend again until smooth.
4. Pour into a glass and serve.

Nutritional Info (per serving):

- Calories: 150
- Protein: 2g
- Carbohydrates: 35g
- Fat: 1g
- Fiber: 5g

Cook Time: None **Prep Time:** 5 minutes *Servings:* 1

Avocado and Spinach Smoothie

Ingredients:

- 1/2 avocado

- 1 cup spinach

- 1/2 banana

- 1/2 cup almond milk

- 1 tablespoon honey or maple syrup

Instructions:

1. Place avocado, spinach, banana, almond milk, and honey or maple syrup in a blender.

2. Blend until smooth.

3. Pour into a glass and serve.

Nutritional Info (per serving):

- Calories: 200

- Protein: 4g

- Carbohydrates: 25g

- Fat: 11g

- Fiber: 7g

Cook Time: None **Prep Time:** 5 minutes *Servings:* 1

Blueberry and Chia Smoothie

Ingredients:

- 1/2 cup blueberries
- 1/2 banana
- 1 tablespoon chia seeds
- 1 cup almond milk
- 1 tablespoon honey or maple syrup

Instructions:

1. Place blueberries, banana, chia seeds, almond milk, and honey or maple syrup in a blender.
2. Blend until smooth.
3. Pour into a glass and serve.

Nutritional Info (per serving):

- Calories: 200
- Protein: 4g
- Carbohydrates: 35g
- Fat: 6g
- Fiber: 9g

Cook Time: None **Prep Time:** 5 minutes *Servings:* 1

Blueberry and Chia Smoothie

Raw Cacao and Banana Smoothie

Ingredients:

- 1 tablespoon raw cacao powder

- 1/2 banana

- 1 cup almond milk

- 1 tablespoon almond butter

- 1 tablespoon honey or maple syrup

Instructions:

1. Place raw cacao powder, banana, almond milk, almond butter, and honey or maple syrup in a blender.

2. Blend until smooth.

3. Pour into a glass and serve.

Nutritional Info (per serving):

- Calories: 250

- Protein: 6g

- Carbohydrates: 30g

- Fat: 13g

- Fiber: 7g

Cook Time: None **Prep Time:** 5 minutes *Servings:* 1

Kale and Apple Smoothie

Ingredients:

- 1 cup kale leaves, stems removed
- 1/2 green apple, cored and chopped
- 1/2 banana
- 1/2 cup coconut water
- 1 tablespoon lemon juice
- Ice cubes (optional)

Instructions:

1. Place kale leaves, apple, banana, coconut water, and lemon juice in a blender.
2. Blend until smooth.
3. Add ice cubes if desired and blend again until smooth.
4. Pour into a glass and serve.

Nutritional Info (per serving):

- Calories: 100
- Protein: 3g
- Carbohydrates: 25g
- Fat: 1g
- Fiber: 6g

Cook Time: None **Prep Time:** 5 minutes *Servings:* 1

Strawberry and Coconut Smoothie

Ingredients:

- 1/2 cup strawberries

- 1/2 banana

- 1/2 cup coconut milk

- 1 tablespoon shredded coconut

- 1 tablespoon honey or maple syrup

Instructions:

1. Place strawberries, banana, coconut milk, shredded coconut, and honey or maple syrup in a blender.

2. Blend until smooth.

3. Pour into a glass and serve.

Nutritional Info (per serving):

- Calories: 200

- Protein: 2g

- Carbohydrates: 30g

- Fat: 9g

- Fiber: 5g

Cook Time: None **Prep Time:** 5 minutes *Servings:* 1

Spirulina and Pineapple Smoothie

Ingredients:

- 1/2 teaspoon spirulina powder

- 1/2 cup pineapple chunks

- 1/2 banana

- 1/2 cup coconut water

- 1 tablespoon honey or maple syrup

Instructions:

1. Place spirulina powder, pineapple chunks, banana, coconut water, and honey or maple syrup in a blender.

2. Blend until smooth.

3. Pour into a glass and serve.

Nutritional Info (per serving):

- Calories: 150

- Protein: 2g

- Carbohydrates: 35g

- Fat: 1g

- Fiber: 4g

Cook Time: None *Prep Time:* 5 minutes *Servings:* 1

Raw Carrot and Ginger Smoothie

Ingredients:

- 1/2 cup chopped carrots

- 1/2 banana

- 1 tablespoon fresh ginger, peeled and chopped

- 1 cup coconut water

- 1 tablespoon lemon juice

- Ice cubes (optional)

Instructions:

1. Place chopped carrots, banana, ginger, coconut water, and lemon juice in a blender.

2. Blend until smooth.

3. Add ice cubes if desired and blend again until smooth.

4. Pour into a glass and serve.

Nutritional Info (per serving):

- Calories: 100

- Protein: 2g

- Carbohydrates: 25g

- Fat: 0g

- Fiber: 5g

Cook Time: None **Prep Time:** 5 minutes *Servings:* 1

Beet and Berry Smoothie

Ingredients:

- 1/2 cup chopped beets
- 1/2 cup mixed berries (such as strawberries, raspberries, and blueberries)
- 1/2 banana
- 1 cup almond milk
- 1 tablespoon honey or maple syrup

Instructions:

1. Place chopped beets, mixed berries, banana, almond milk, and honey or maple syrup in a blender.
2. Blend until smooth.
3. Pour into a glass and serve.

Nutritional Info (per serving):

- Calories: 150
- Protein: 3g
- Carbohydrates: 30g
- Fat: 3g
- Fiber: 8g

Cook Time: None **Prep Time:** 5 minutes *Servings:* 1

Almond Butter and Banana Smoothie

Ingredients:

- 1 tablespoon almond butter
- 1/2 banana
- 1 cup almond milk
- 1 tablespoon honey or maple syrup
- 1/2 teaspoon cinnamon

Instructions:

1. Place almond butter, banana, almond milk, honey or maple syrup, and cinnamon in a blender.
2. Blend until smooth.
3. Pour into a glass and serve.

Nutritional Info (per serving):

- Calories: 250
- Protein: 6g
- Carbohydrates: 30g
- Fat: 13g
- Fiber: 7g

Cook Time: None **Prep Time:** 5 minutes *Servings:* 1

Cucumber and Mint Smoothie

Ingredients:

- 1/2 cucumber, peeled and chopped

- 1/4 cup fresh mint leaves

- 1/2 green apple, cored and chopped

- 1/2 lemon, juiced

- 1 cup coconut water

- Ice cubes (optional)

Instructions:

1. Place cucumber, mint leaves, green apple, lemon juice, coconut water, and ice cubes in a blender.

2. Blend until smooth.

3. Pour into a glass and serve.

Nutritional Info (per serving):

- Calories: 70

- Protein: 2g

- Carbohydrates: 18g

- Fat: 1g

- Fiber: 4g

Cook Time: None **Prep Time:** 5 minutes *Servings:* 1

Raw Green Apple and Celery Smoothie

Ingredients:

- 1/2 green apple, cored and chopped
- 2 celery stalks, chopped
- 1/2 cucumber, peeled and chopped
- 1/2 lemon, juiced
- 1 cup coconut water
- Ice cubes (optional)

Instructions:

1. Place green apple, celery stalks, cucumber, lemon juice, coconut water, and ice cubes in a blender.
2. Blend until smooth.
3. Pour into a glass and serve.

Nutritional Info (per serving):

- Calories: 70
- Protein: 2g
- Carbohydrates: 18g
- Fat: 1g
- Fiber: 4g

Cook Time: None **Prep Time:** 5 minutes *Servings:* 1

Turmeric and Orange Smoothie

Ingredients:

- 1/2 teaspoon ground turmeric
- 1 orange, peeled and segmented
- 1/2 banana
- 1/2 cup almond milk
- 1 tablespoon honey or maple syrup

Instructions:

1. Place ground turmeric, orange segments, banana, almond milk, and honey or maple syrup in a blender.
2. Blend until smooth.
3. Pour into a glass and serve.

Nutritional Info (per serving):

- Calories: 150
- Protein: 3g
- Carbohydrates: 35g
- Fat: 2g
- Fiber: 6g

Cook Time: None **Prep Time:** 5 minutes *Servings:* 1

Raspberry and Lemon Smoothie

Ingredients:

- 1/2 cup raspberries
- 1/2 banana
- 1/2 lemon, juiced
- 1 cup almond milk
- 1 tablespoon honey or maple syrup

Instructions:

1. Place raspberries, banana, lemon juice, almond milk, and honey or maple syrup in a blender.
2. Blend until smooth.
3. Pour into a glass and serve.

Nutritional Info (per serving):

- Calories: 150
- Protein: 3g
- Carbohydrates: 30g
- Fat: 3g
- Fiber: 8g

Cook Time: None **Prep Time:** 5 minutes *Servings:* 1

Coconut Water and Berry Smoothie

Ingredients:

- 1/2 cup mixed berries (such as strawberries, blueberries, and raspberries)

- 1/2 banana

- 1/2 cup coconut water

- 1 tablespoon chia seeds

- 1 tablespoon honey or maple syrup

Instructions:

1. Place mixed berries, banana, coconut water, chia seeds, and honey or maple syrup in a blender.

2. Blend until smooth.

3. Pour into a glass and serve.

Nutritional Info (per serving):

- Calories: 150

- Protein: 3g

- Carbohydrates: 30g

- Fat: 3g

- Fiber: 8g

Cook Time: None **Prep Time:** 5 minutes *Servings:* 1

Ginger and Pear Smoothie

Ingredients:

- 1 pear, cored and chopped

- 1/2 inch fresh ginger, peeled and chopped

- 1/2 banana

- 1 cup almond milk

- 1 tablespoon honey or maple syrup

Instructions:

1. Place pear, ginger, banana, almond milk, and honey or maple syrup in a blender.

2. Blend until smooth.

3. Pour into a glass and serve.

Nutritional Info (per serving):

- Calories: 150

- Protein: 3g

- Carbohydrates: 30g

- Fat: 3g

- Fiber: 8g

Cook Time: None **Prep Time:** 5 minutes *Servings:* 1

Raw Spinach and Avocado Smoothie

Ingredients:

- 1 cup spinach

- 1/2 avocado

- 1/2 banana

- 1 cup coconut water

- 1 tablespoon lemon juice

Instructions:

1. Place spinach, avocado, banana, coconut water, and lemon juice in a blender.

2. Blend until smooth.

3. Pour into a glass and serve.

Nutritional Info (per serving):

- Calories: 200

- Protein: 4g

- Carbohydrates: 25g

- Fat: 12g

- Fiber: 7g

Cook Time: None **Prep Time:** 5 minutes *Servings:* 1

Mango and Coconut Smoothie

Ingredients:

- 1/2 cup chopped mango

- 1/2 banana

- 1/2 cup coconut milk

- 1 tablespoon shredded coconut

- 1 tablespoon honey or maple syrup

Instructions:

1. Place mango, banana, coconut milk, shredded coconut, and honey or maple syrup in a blender.

2. Blend until smooth.

3. Pour into a glass and serve.

Nutritional Info (per serving):

- Calories: 200

- Protein: 3g

- Carbohydrates: 35g

- Fat: 7g

- Fiber: 5g

Cook Time: None **Prep Time:** 5 minutes *Servings:* 1

Raw Red Pepper and Tomato Smoothie

Ingredients:

- 1/2 red pepper, seeded and chopped
- 1 tomato, chopped
- 1/2 cucumber, peeled and chopped
- 1/2 lemon, juiced
- 1 cup coconut water
- Ice cubes (optional)

Instructions:

1. Place red pepper, tomato, cucumber, lemon juice, coconut water, and ice cubes in a blender.
2. Blend until smooth.
3. Pour into a glass and serve.

Nutritional Info (per serving):

- Calories: 100
- Protein: 2g
- Carbohydrates: 20g
- Fat: 1g
- Fiber: 5g

Cook Time: None **Prep Time:** 5 minutes *Servings:* 1

Pineapple and Kale Smoothie

Ingredients:

- 1/2 cup chopped pineapple

- 1 cup kale leaves, stems removed

- 1/2 banana

- 1/2 cup coconut water

- 1 tablespoon honey or maple syrup

Instructions:

1. Place pineapple, kale leaves, banana, coconut water, and honey or maple syrup in a blender.

2. Blend until smooth.

3. Pour into a glass and serve.

Nutritional Info (per serving):

- Calories: 150

- Protein: 3g

- Carbohydrates: 30g

- Fat: 1g

- Fiber: 6g

Cook Time: None **Prep Time:** 5 minutes *Servings:* 1

Raw Broccoli and Apple Smoothie

Ingredients:

- 1/2 cup chopped broccoli

- 1/2 apple, cored and chopped

- 1/2 banana

- 1 cup almond milk

- 1 tablespoon honey or maple syrup

Instructions:

1. Place broccoli, apple, banana, almond milk, and honey or maple syrup in a blender.

2. Blend until smooth.

3. Pour into a glass and serve.

Nutritional Info (per serving):

- Calories: 150

- Protein: 3g

- Carbohydrates: 30g

- Fat: 3g

- Fiber: 8g

Cook Time: None **Prep Time:** 5 minutes *Servings:* 1

Papaya and Lime Smoothie

Ingredients:

- 1/2 cup chopped papaya
- 1/2 banana
- 1/2 lime, juiced
- 1 cup coconut water
- 1 tablespoon honey or maple syrup

Instructions:

1. Place papaya, banana, lime juice, coconut water, and honey or maple syrup in a blender.
2. Blend until smooth.
3. Pour into a glass and serve.

Nutritional Info (per serving):

- Calories: 150
- Protein: 3g
- Carbohydrates: 30g
- Fat: 3g
- Fiber: 8g

Cook Time: None **Prep Time:** 5 minutes *Servings:* 1

Raw Cucumber and Pineapple Smoothie

Ingredients:

- 1/2 cucumber, peeled and chopped

- 1/2 cup chopped pineapple

- 1/2 banana

- 1 cup coconut water

- 1 tablespoon fresh mint leaves

Instructions:

1. Place cucumber, pineapple, banana, coconut water, and fresh mint leaves in a blender.

2. Blend until smooth.

3. Pour into a glass and serve.

Nutritional Info (per serving):

- Calories: 120

- Protein: 2g

- Carbohydrates: 29g

- Fat: 1g

- Fiber: 4g

Cook Time: None **Prep Time:** 5 minutes *Servings:* 1

Raw Pumpkin Seed and Banana Smoothie

Ingredients:

- 1 tablespoon raw pumpkin seeds

- 1 banana

- 1 cup almond milk

- 1 tablespoon honey or maple syrup

- 1/2 teaspoon cinnamon

Instructions:

1. Place raw pumpkin seeds, banana, almond milk, honey or maple syrup, and cinnamon in a blender.

2. Blend until smooth.

3. Pour into a glass and serve.

Nutritional Info (per serving):

- Calories: 200

- Protein: 5g

- Carbohydrates: 35g

- Fat: 6g

- Fiber: 4g

Cook Time: None **Prep Time:** 5 minutes *Servings:* 1

Raw Carrot and Orange Smoothie

Ingredients:

- 1/2 cup chopped carrots

- 1 orange, peeled and segmented

- 1/2 banana

- 1 cup coconut water

- 1 tablespoon lemon juice

Instructions:

1. Place chopped carrots, orange segments, banana, coconut water, and lemon juice in a blender.

2. Blend until smooth.

3. Pour into a glass and serve.

Nutritional Info (per serving):

- Calories: 120

- Protein: 2g

- Carbohydrates: 30g

- Fat: 0g

- Fiber: 6g

Cook Time: None **Prep Time:** 5 minutes *Servings:* 1

Apple and Cinnamon Smoothie

Ingredients:

- 1 apple, cored and chopped

- 1/2 banana

- 1 cup almond milk

- 1/2 teaspoon cinnamon

- 1 tablespoon honey or maple syrup

Instructions:

1. Place apple, banana, almond milk, cinnamon, and honey or maple syrup in a blender.

2. Blend until smooth.

3. Pour into a glass and serve.

Nutritional Info (per serving):

- Calories: 150

- Protein: 3g

- Carbohydrates: 35g

- Fat: 2g

- Fiber: 6g

Cook Time: None **Prep Time:** 5 minutes *Servings:* 1

Raw Hemp Seed and Berry Smoothie

Ingredients:

- 1 tablespoon hemp seeds
- 1/2 cup mixed berries (such as strawberries, blueberries, and raspberries)
- 1/2 banana
- 1 cup almond milk
- 1 tablespoon honey or maple syrup

Instructions:

1. Place hemp seeds, mixed berries, banana, almond milk, and honey or maple syrup in a blender.
2. Blend until smooth.
3. Pour into a glass and serve.

Nutritional Info (per serving):

- Calories: 180
- Protein: 5g
- Carbohydrates: 30g
- Fat: 7g
- Fiber: 6g

Cook Time: None **Prep Time:** 5 minutes *Servings:* 1

Raw Watermelon and Basil Smoothie

Ingredients:

- 1 cup chopped watermelon

- 1/2 banana

- 1/2 cup coconut water

- 1 tablespoon fresh basil leaves

- 1 tablespoon lime juice

Instructions:

1. Place chopped watermelon, banana, coconut water, fresh basil leaves, and lime juice in a blender.

2. Blend until smooth.

3. Pour into a glass and serve.

Nutritional Info (per serving):

- Calories: 90

- Protein: 1g

- Carbohydrates: 22g

- Fat: 0g

- Fiber: 2g

Cook Time: None **Prep Time:** 5 minutes *Servings:* 1